AF333587

DISSEMINATED INTRAVASCULAR COAGULATION (DIC)

CLINICAL MANIFESTATIONS, DIAGNOSIS AND TREATMENT OPTIONS

RECENT ADVANCES IN HEMATOLOGY RESEARCH

Additional books in this series can be found on Nova's website
under the Series tab.

Additional e-books in this series can be found on Nova's website
under the e-book tab.

DISSEMINATED INTRAVASCULAR COAGULATION (DIC)

CLINICAL MANIFESTATIONS, DIAGNOSIS AND TREATMENT OPTIONS

BALWINDER SINGH, M.D.

EDITOR

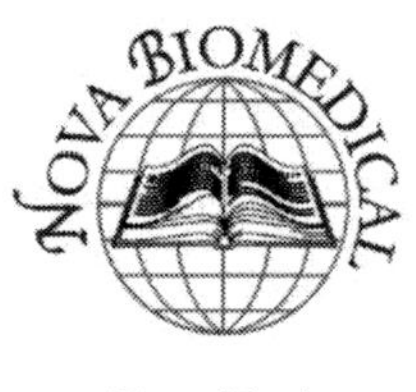

New York

Library of Congress Cataloging-in-Publication Data

ISBN: 978-1-62948-323-8

Library of Congress Control Number: 2013950460

Published by Nova Science Publishers, Inc. † New York

Contents

Preface

Disseminated Intravascular Coagulation is a devastating syndrome characterized by the systemic activation of widespread activation of the coagulation cascade and thrombosis, which may result in severe bleeding and may lead to organ failure. Recent studies have shown that the incidence of DIC is decreasing, especially in men. Despite the improvements in health care delivery, the morbidity and mortality due to DIC remains very high. Early diagnosis and accurate prognosis are important in improving the outcomes of patients with DIC.

However, there is a lack of a gold standard diagnostic test to diagnose DIC and there is a scarcity of treatment or management strategies. Therefore, an understanding of the pathophysiology, ability to diagnose the DIC syndrome and to treat early, is the key. This book provides an important timely update on the clinical manifestations, important risk factors, and treatment strategies for DIC, and provides in-depth information on pathophysiological aspects and various diagnostic scores used to diagnose DIC. Furthermore, we focused on certain important factors related to DIC such as Sepsis, chronic DIC in cancer patients, coagulopathy of liver disorders vs DIC, and DIC in urological malignancies.

In addition, this book provides evidence from an important study determining the predictors influencing the hospital mortality rates of the critically ill patients with DIC. This book offers a wide scope of information for physicians in all fields, whether they are intensivists, primary care physicians or oncologists, this will be an important source for identifying the DIC syndrome early, and the appropriate steps to improve patient outcomes will be taken sooner.

I would like to thank all the contributing authors from different fields, who have made a sincere effort to provide in-depth knowledge of DIC in various different settings. I hope that this book would be able to impart important knowledge and understanding on this serious syndrome and help the physicians to diagnose and manage DIC appropriately.

In: Disseminated Intravascular Coagulation (DIC)   ISBN: 978-1-62948-323-8
Editor: Balwinder Singh   © 2014 Nova Science Publishers, Inc.

Chapter I

Disseminated Intravascular Coagulation: Clinical Manifestations

Akhilesh Kumar Tiwari, MD[1], Michell Gulabani, MD[2],
Prashant Dass, MD[3] and Rishi Raj Sanjay, MD[2]*

[1]Department of Anaesthesia and Critical Care,
National University Hospital, Singapore.
[2]Department of Anaesthesia and Critical Care,
Batra Hospital and Medical Research Centre, New Delhi, India
[3]Department of Pharmacology, M R Medical College,
Gulbarga, Karnataka, India

Abstract

Disseminated intravascular coagulation is a disorder found to be associated with a number of underlying predisposing factors. It has come to be known by various names such as consumption coagulopathy, defibrination among various others. DIC; however, is the most widely used and accepted. The grave prognosis of DIC warrants an early

---

* Corresponding Author address: Dr. Akhilesh KumarTiwari, National University Hospial, 5 Lower Kent Ridge Road, Singapore. Email:draktiwari11@gmail.com.

diagnosis and prompt management. To achieve this, clinicians should have in-depth knowledge of underlying predisposing factors, clinical features and laboratory diagnostic protocols. The present chapter will focus mainly on the clinical features which are very variable, ranging from severe hemorrhagic manifestation in acute cases of DIC to sub-clinical thrombotic episode in patients suffering from chronic DIC.

Keywords: Disseminated Intravascular coagulation, consumptioncoagulo-pathy, Waterhouse-Friderichsen syndrome, Trousseau syndrome

Introduction

Disseminated Intravascular Coagulation (DIC) is an acquired syndrome, associated with various underlying disorders such as sepsis, malignancy, haematological disorders, trauma and obstetric conditions [1-3]. In an acute setting it is a potentially fatal and rapidly progressive disorder, mandating a prompt diagnosis and rapid treatment; whereas, at the same time in a sub-acute or chronic setting it has a very indolent course and often may be overlooked due to normal or near normal hematological and coagulation profile. This condition is associated with widespread activation of coagulation system leading to multiple organ dysfunction syndrome (MODS) which is either ischaemic or inflammatory in origin [4]. This condition is associated with combination of both thrombosis and hemorrhage, and due to its potentially fatal nature it has also been referred as "Malignant syndrome." [5]

DIC is never a primary disorder and is almost always associated with an underlying condition the details of which have been discussed in a different chapter. DIC tends to occur in about 1% of all the hospital admission [6]. The main symptoms of bleeding and thrombosis and the consequences thereof depends on the underlying cause and the rapidity with which it progresses. There are two main clinical forms which have been described: acute and chronic; although, a lot of overlap exists between these two entities. We will initially be concentrating upon two clinical forms of DIC: acute and chronic . One should always remember that it is the underlying process which dominates the clinical presentation in most of the acute DIC cases.In cases of chronic DIC the initial presentation may not be of the underlying disorder.Thrombosis involving both arteries and veins have often been observed in these patients.

The clinical manifestation is variable, with symptoms arising either due to hypercoagulable state or hemorrhagic tendency. The clinical course of the patient suffering from DIC can be further subdivided into [7]:

1) Stage of hypercoagulability.
2) Stage of exhaustion (Consumption coagulopathy)
3) Hyperfibrinolysis.

Acute DIC

Acute DIC has fulminant course, developing in conditions which are associated with massive release of tissue factor leading to explosive generation of thrombin. The fulminant nature of acute DIC is because the consumption coagulopathy is way ahead of the capacity of the liver to synthesize coagulation factors, and bone marrow to produce platelets. This leads to massive bleeding tendency, which is potentially lethal and evolves over period of hours to days. The common conditions associated with acute DIC are sepsis, trauma, shock, peri-operative states, certain obstetric conditions and should always be regarded and treated as medical emergency

Chronic DIC

Chronic DIC usually runs an indolent and subtle course and takes months to progress. The laboratory parameters used to diagnose acute DIC may be normal or near normal in these clinical scenarios. Chronic DIC arises due to presence of chronic low grade persistent stimulation of intravascular coagulation as observed in cases such as retained dead fetus, subdural hematoma [8, 9], post-biopsy renal hematoma [10], carcinomatosis, aortic aneurysm, giant haemangiomas [11]. Rarely chronic DIC has also shown to manifest itself as a renal mass mimicking Wilm's tumour [12]. In these conditions the counter regulatory mechanism of the body is effective to prevent the rapid progression of disease as a result of which the laboratory values are not diagnostic as in cases of acute DIC. Malignancy is often associated with chronic DIC, but certain malignancies like acute promyelocytic leukemia (APL) may lead to acute DIC.

Table 1. Enumerates important differentiating point between both acute and chronic DIC

	Acute DIC	**Chronic DIC**
Etiology	Septicemia (Gram positive, negative, viral, fungal, protozoal, e.t.c.), acute obstetric complications, acute tissue injury	Malignancies, connective tissue disorders, chronic infections, haemangioma, retained dead fetus
Clinical course	Hours to days	Months
Clinical features	External and internal bleeding, easy bruisabiity, Ischemia infarction and inflammation leading to MODS	Superficial and Deep vein thrombosis, Trousseau syndrome among few notable ones
Laboratory parameters	Prothrombin time (PT), activated partial thromboplastin time, D-Dimer, Thrombin time, fibrinogen level, fibrinogen degradation products along with the presence of fragmented red cells in the peripheral smear is sufficient enough to make a diagnosis.	They may be normal to near normal

Table 2 enumerates the common symptoms which a patient suffering from DIC may have [13].

Table 2. Common clinical manifestation of DIC

Symptom	**Incidence (%)**
Bleeding	64
Renal Dysfunction	25
Hepatic dysfunction	19
Pulmonary Manifestation	16
Shock	14
Thrombosis	7
Neurological impairment	2

We will now be discussing the common symptoms observed in patients suffering from DIC.

Bleeding

Bleeding manifestation in DICis variable, and may range from small petechiae to massive internal or external bleeding. External bleeding can be in the form of persistent oozing from cannulation, surgical or tissue injury sites. Internal bleeding can be within the serous cavities of the body or in the form of intra-cranial hemorrhage. Patients having bleeding manifestations due to DIC usually have grave prognosis, and the body, often cannot compensate for this stage of consumptive coagulopathy. This clinical course has often been referred to as "Overt syndrome/DIC." [7] Patient may start to have hematuria, and in cases of bleeding into gastrointestinal tract the patients may have black tarry stools, blood in nasogastric tube, hematemesis, abdominal pain and distension along with absent or hyper-active bowel sounds. Black tarry stool occurring in these patients have also been implicated to extensive necrosis of the colon known as "terminal hemorrhagic necrotizing enteropathy." [14] Focal neurological deficits should raise the suspicion towards possible intracranial hemorrhage in susceptible individuals. Patients with chronic DIC usually exhibit minor skin and mucosal bleeding.

Profuse bleeding from three different sites which may be unrelated is not uncommon especially in acute form of DIC.

Renal Dysfunction

Kidneys are one of the commonest organ system affected. Renal faiure and the consequent complications have been reported in the literature in established cases of DIC. Renal failure; however, presenting as a sign of DIC is extremely rare [15]. The possible mechanism of renal injury in patients suffering from DIC is microthombus formation in afferent arterioles and lumina of glomerular capillary. Complete blockage of these afferent arterioles often leads to "Bloodless Glomeruli." Other possible mechanism of renal dysfunction in these patients is secondary to circulatory collapse, which leads to renal hypo-perfusion, acute tubular necrosis (ATN) and acute renal failure (ARF) [16].

Hepatic Dysfunction

Liver is the seat of coagulation factor synthesis. Hepatic dysfunction and DIC are closely inter-related. Mechanism of hepatic dysfunction in patients suffering from DIC is essentially the same, i.e., microvasular thrombosis in small and medium sized vessels involving both arteries and veins. Marked elevation of serum bilirubin and hepatic enzymes is a sign of multiple thrombi in the liver [14]. Other possible causes of hepatocellular injury in these patients are sepsis and circulatory collapse. Thrombotic events as observed in DIC and other diseases is seen to occur mainly in portal and mesentric veins [17]. DIC and decompensated cirrhosis usually have similar coagulation abnormality [17]; however, with the availability of newer diagnostic tools like prothrombin fragment F1+2 fibrinopeptide A, soluble fibrin, D-Dimer, thrombinantithrombin complex (TAT) and plasmin α_2 antiplasmin complex have led to a newer clinical entity known as accelerated intravascular coagulation and fibrinolysis (AICF) [18]. AICF was previously defined as low-grade DIC, but point worth noting is that patients suffering from AICF and liver cirrhosis are at higher risk of developing "overt DIC." Development of jaundice in patients suffering from DIC is found to be more common in patients with an underlying septic etiology [19].

Pulmonary Manifestations

Pulmonary manifestation is observed in about 16% of the patients suffering from DIC. This presentation may be in the form of pulmonary hemorrhagic syndrome [20], pulmonary infarction or myocardial infarction [21]. The common symptoms observed in this scenario is dyspnoea, chest pain and hemoptysis and the physical examination may reveal wheeze, rhonchi and pleural friction rub. Radiological investigations performed may reveal intra-alveolar hemorrhage. The underlying mechanism of the pulmonary manifestation is again the same, with damage to vascular endothelium being one of the mechanism. Pulmonary manifestation also arises secondary to the underlying cause responsible for DIC. Development of ARDS and ALI in cases of sepsis in one such example.

Shock and Circulatory Arrest

Shock and ultimately circulatory arrest in patients sufering from DIC is multifactorial. Few of the proposed mechanism are: hypovolemia due to bleeding, vasular obstruction of microvessels due to thrombi formation and increased vasular permeablity due to fibrin degradation products, kinins, histamine and other inflammatory cytokines, which further leads to decreased intravascular volume due to extravasation of fluid from blood vessels.

Thrombosis

The common thrombotic manifestation in patients suffering from DIC are necrotic skin lesions [22], pulmonary thromboembolism, limb ischemia, cerebral and coronary thrombosis [19]. These necrotic and gangrenous lesions may also be associated with tachycadia and fever. Similar thrombotic mechanism has also been observed in patients suffering from various malignancies. First association of thrombosis with malignancy was reported in the year 1865 by Trousseau [23, 24], and was thought to be because of underlying coagulopathy. Common malignancies associated with the development of this syndrome are pancreatic, lung and ovarian [24-26]. Histologically mucin producing adenocarcinomas are the ones which are responsible for this syndrome [27]. Mucin produced by certain adenocarcinomas has been thought to be responsible for platelet aggregation [28].

Neurological Dysfunction

DIC could be one of the implicating factor responsible for stroke in patients with malignancy. Few of the common neurological complications which these patients may suffer are vascular occlusion, coma, seizures, hemiparesis subarachnoid hemorrhage along with multiple hemorrhage and infarct [29]. Central neurological manifestations are more common than peripheral symptoms. Thrombosis of vasa nervosum and consequent ischemia of the nerves have been linked to the development of peripheral neuropathy in children suffering from diabetic ketoacidosis complicated by DIC [30]. Severity of neurological manifestation in DIC depends on the type, site and severity of the thrombotic and hemorrhagic lesions. Matsuda in his paper [14] further proposed the classification of DIC into two main type based on the underlying clinical manifestations. The one with the predominant bleeding manifestations were labelled as "Fibrinolysis dominant DIC" and acute promyelocytic leukemia is one such example leading to this variant. Conditions such as sepsis, on the other hand, is associated with severe organ dysfunction and this variant is labelled as "Coagulation dominant type." Bleeding manifestations arising in the latter are usually not severe and have been blamed to bebecause of thrombocytopenia [14]. The ideal diagnostic algorithm for DIC should have a different set of criteria for each identifiable underlying cause, which, although is not practicable. Scientific and Standardization Committee (SSC) of the International Society on Thrombosis and Haemostasis (ISTH) have proposed the classification of DIC into overt and non-overt and proposed a set of guidelines for the same [31]. Few authorities; however, are of the opinion that these criteria are not diagnostic; rather they should be used for initiating treatment. Detailed discussion of these guidelines is beyond the scope of the current chapter and is to be discussed in a separate chapter. We will now discuss few salient points of certain important etiological factors associated with DIC:

DIC and Sepsis

Sepsis is one of the leading causes of mortality [32], and DIC have been often found to complicate the issue [33-35]. Overt DIC can be found in about 25-50% of cases and if found associated, have high mortality. One of the most severe clinical manifestations of DIC is Purpura Fulminans [36]. It is a condition encountered in newborns and infants, and is represented by extensive skin necrosis over buttocks and extremities. PurpuraFulminans usually occurs 3-4 weeks after mild viral infections such as rubella, varicella, etc., NPF have also been reported to be occurring in patients with protein C deficiency [37]. Patients with underlying sepsis may have variable manifestations ranging from thromboembolic phenomenon to micro-vascular fibrin deposition leading to MODS [38]. They may also present with severe bleeding manifestation; however, it is not surprising to find patients with sepsis to have combination of both bleeding and thrombotic manifestation. "Waterhouse-Friderichsen syndrome" (adrenal haemorrhage) is one such example reported often in meningococcal septicaemia, and has a mortality rate of 55-60% [39]. Sepsis induced DIC is particularly more common in immunocompromised and asplenic patients.

DIC and Tissue Trauma

Tissue trauma due to any cause like road traffic accidents, war injuries, burns, heat stroke, major surgeries and traumatic brain injuries have been associated with DIC. The biopsied specimen of brain, liver, lungs, kidneys, pancreas and liver have all shown the presence of microthrombus in the vasculature in trauma patients.

Heat strokes have also been associated with DIC, with the presence of fibrin and hemorrhagic infarcts. The patients with heat stroke have been found to be having a very high-level of serum interleukins 6 and 8 [40]. Clinical severity of heat stroke has a positive correlation with the degree of inflammation and stimulation of coagulation pathway.

DIC in Obstetrics

Pregnancy in itself is a hypercoagulable condition which in the presence of certain clinical conditions like abruptio placenta, eclampsia, hydatidiform mole, prolonged shock and intrauterine fetal demise lead to DIC. Abruptio placenta is the most frequent obstetric condition associated with coagulation failure and may be seen in apparently healthy individuals or in cases suffering from pre-eclampsia [22]. Only about 10% of pregnant females sufering from abruptio placenta have significant coagulation abnormalities [41]. Patients who suffer from only minor degree of abruption may deliver a normal healthy baby. In severe cases patient may go into hypovolemic shock with almost about five litres of concelaed blood loss [22]. Persistent oozing from the venepuncture sites, easy bruisability, nasal or oral bleed should raise the suspicion of an underlying DIC, and prompt screening test should be immediately undertaken.

DIC in Malignancy

Patients with solid tumours and mucin producing adenocarcinomas with additional risk factors like advancing age, stage of the tumour, chemotherapy are at particularly higher risk of DIC. Presence of additional risk factors like septicemia, prolonged immobilization and secondaries in the liver increases the likelihood of developing DIC. Presence of arterial or venous thrombosis, pulmonary thromboembolism, superficial and deep vein thrombosis have been regularly reported in literature in patients suffering from malignant tumour [42, 43]. Trousseau syndrome as discussed above is one such manifestation and is associated with poor prognosis [44]. Patients with malignancy may suffer from both acute and chronic form of DIC.

General features relevant to abnormal coagulopahty like prolonged oozing is often reported. Microvascular thrombosis \in the skin may present as petechiae, acral cyanosis, gangrene of digits, nose and ear lobules. These gangrenous changes are most often observed in the areas of end artery circulation [45]. Organ dysfunction is very common in these patients; however, at times it may also be beacuse of the underlying malignancy itself and the differentiation may be difficult. Organ system commonly found to be affected include lungs, kidneys, central nervous system with other sites where traces of microthrombi have been found include heart, pancreas, kidneys and testes [45]. Chronic form of DIC as discussed already runs a subclinical course and Trousseau syndrome is one such manifestation.

Conclusion

In the present chapter, we had directed our focus on the clinical manifestations of DIC, with a brief dicsussion on the important etiological factors. In majority of the patients, the clinical picture is a reflection of the underlying disease process. The clinical manifestations of DIC are highly variable and are determined by factors like etiology, severity and duration of the underlying pathology. Due to the grave prognosis, which DIC has, it has aptly been called as "Death is coming." [46]

References

[1]   Levi M, Ten Cate H. Disseminated intravascular coagulation. *N Engl J Med* 1999; 341:586-592,

[2]   Muller-Berghaus G, ten Cate H, Levi M. Disseminated intravascular coagulation: clinical spectrum and established as well as new diagnostic approaches. *Thromb Haemost* 1999;82:706–12.

[3]   Levi M, de Jonge E, van der Poll T, ten Cate H. Advances in the understanding of the pathogenetic pathways of disseminated

intravascular coagulation result in more insight in the clinical picture and better management strategies. *SeminThrombHemost* 2001; 27:569–75.

[4]   Levi M. Disseminated intravascular coagulation. *Crit Care Med* 2007;35:2191–5.

[5]   Ph. Cauchie, Ch. Cauchie, K. ZouaouiBoudjeltia, E. Carlier, N. Deschepper, D. Govaerts, M. Migaud-Fressart, B. Woodhams, and D. Brohe′e. Diagnosis and prognosis of overt disseminated intravascular coagulation in a general hospital – Meaning of the ISTH score system, Fibrin monomers, and Lipoprotein- C – Reactive Protein Complex formation *American Journal of Hematology* 81:414–419 2006.

[6]   Matsuda T. Clinical aspects of DIC--disseminated intravascular coagulation. *Pol J Pharmacol*1996; 48:73.

[7]   Urge J, Strojil J. Early diagnosis of DIC development into the overt phase. Biomed Pap Med FacUnivPalacky Olomouc Czech Repub. 2006 Nov;150(2):267-9.

[8]   Pollak L, Schiffer J, Leonov Y et al. Acute subdural hematoma following disseminated intravascular coagulation associated with an obstetric catastrophe. *Isr J Med Sci* 1995; 31: 489-91.

[9]   Ng PC, Fok TF, Lee CH et al. Massive subdural hematoma: An unusual complication of septicemia in preterm very low birth weight infants. *J Paediatr Child Health* 1998; 34: 296-8.

[10]   Dara T, Lohr J. Disseminated Intravascular Coagulation following percutaneous renal biopsy. *Am J Nephrol* 1991; 11: 343-4.

[11]   Baglin T. Fortnightly review: Disseminated intravascular coagulation: Diagnosis and treatment. *BMJ* 1996; 312:683-7.

[12]   Somashekhar M, Kadamba PS, Wakodkar M. Chronic disseminated intravascular coagulation presenting as renal mass. *J Indian AssocPediatrSurg* Oct-Dec 2008; 13.4: 144-146.

[13]   Bope& Kellerman: Conn's Current Therapy 2013, 1st ed. 2012 Saunders. Chapter 13: *Hematology*. 793-795.

[14]   Tamotsu Matsuda. Clinical aspect of DIC – Disseminated Intravascular Coagulation. *Pol J Pharmacol.* 1996;48:73-75.

[15]   Ohashi R, Hosokawa Y, Kimura G, Kondo Y, Tanaka K, Tsuchiya S. Acute renal failure as the presenting sign of disseminated intravascular coagulation in a patient with metastatic prostate cancer. *Int J Nephrol Renovasc Dis.* 2013; 6: 47–51.

[16]   http://www.uptodate.com/contents/clinical-features-diagnosis-and-treatment-of-disseminated-intravascular-coagulation-in-adults   accessed on 24th July 2013.

[17] Amitrano L, Guardascione MA, Brancaccio V, Balzano A. Coagulation disorders in liver disease. *Seminars in liver disease* 2002; Vol. 22-1: 83-96.

[18] Joist JH. AICF and DIC in liver cirrhosis: Expressions of a hypercoagulable state. *Am J Gastroenterol* 1999;94:2801–2803.

[19] Siegal T, Seligsohn U, Aghai E, Modan M. Clinical and laboratory aspects of disseminated intravascular coagulation (DIC): a study of 118 cases. *Thromb Haemost.* 1978 Feb 28;39(1):122-34.

[20] Robboy SJ, Minna JD, Colman RW, Birndorf NI, Lopas H. Pulmonary hemorrhage syndrome as a manifestation of disseminated intravascular coagulation: analysis of ten cases. *Chest.* 1973 May;63(5):718-21.

[21] F J Thomson, E W Benbow, R F McMahon, C M Cheshire. Pulmonary infarction, myocardial infarction, and acute disseminated intravascular coagulation. *J ClinPathol.* 1991 December; 44(12): 1034–1036.

[22] Elizabeth A. Letsky. Disseminated intravascular coagulation. *Best practice and Research clinical obstetrics & gynaecology.* Volume 15, Issue 4.623-644.

[23] Trousseau A (1865) Phlegmasiaalbadolens: Clinique medicule de l'Hotel-Dieu de Paris. London. New Sydenham Society.

[24] Takeuchi N, Semba S, Naba K, Maeda T, Tada H, et al. (2013) A Female Presenting with Trousseau Syndrome in End-stage Pancreatic Cancer: A Case Report. 2: 594 doi:10.4172/scientificreports.594.

[25] Sack GH Jr, Levin J, Bell WR (1977) Trousseau's syndrome and other manifestations of chronic disseminated coagulopathy in patients with neoplasms: clinical, pathophysiologic, and therapeutic features. *Medicine* (Baltimore) 56: 1-37.

[26] Cestari DM, Weine DM, Panageas KS, Segal AZ, De Angelis LM (2004) Stroke in patients with cancer: incidence and etiology. *Neurology* 62: 2025-2030.

[27] Sutherland DE, Weitz IC, Liebman HA (2003) Thromboembolic complications of cancer: epidemiology, pathogenesis, diagnosis, and treatment. *Am J Hematol* 72: 43-52.

[28] Wahrenbrock M, Borsig L, Le D, Varki N, Varki A (2003) Selectin-mucin interactions as a probable molecular explanation for the association of Trousseau syndrome with mucinous adenocarcinomas. *J Clin Invest* 112: 853- 862.

[29] Schwartzman RJ, Hill JB. Neurologic complications of disseminated intravascular coagulation. *Neurology.* 1982 Aug;32(8):791-7.

[30] Bonfanti R, Bognetti E, Meschi F, Medaglini S, D'Angelo A, Chiumello G. Disseminated intravascular coagulation and severe peripheral neuropathy complicating ketoacidosis in a newly diagnosed diabetic child. *Acta Diabetol.* 1994 Sep;31(3):173-4.

[31] Kaneko T, Wada H. Diagnostic Criteria and Laboratory Tests for Disseminated Intravascular Coagulation. *J Clin Exp Hematopathol* Vol. 51, No. 2, Nov. 2011. 67-76.

[32] Rangel-Frausto MS, Pittet D, Costigan M, et al. The natural history of the systemic inflammatory response syndrome(SIRS): a prospective study. *JAMA* 1995; 273:117–123.

[33] Gando S, Kameue T, Nanzaki S, et al. Disseminated intravascular coagulation is a frequent complication of systemic inflammatory response syndrome. *ThrombHaemost*1996; 75:224–228

[34] Gando S, Nanzaki S, Kemmotsu O. Disseminated intravascular coagulation and sustained systemic inflammatory response syndrome predict organ dysfunctions after trauma: application of clinical decision analysis. *Ann Surg* 1999; 229:121–127

[35] Wada H, Minamikawa K, Wakita Y, et al. Hemostatic study before onset of disseminated intravascular coagulation. *Am J Hematol* 1993; 43:190–194.

[36] Gerson WT, Dickerman JD, Bovill EG et al. Severe acquired protein C deficiency in purpurafulminans associated with disseminated intravascular coagulation: treatment with protein C concentrate. *Pediatrics* 1993; 91(2): 418-422.

[37] Tiwari AK, Tomar GS, Tayal S, Chadha M, Kapoor MC. Anaesthetic significance and management of a child with neonatal purpurafulminans. *Indian J Anaesth* 2012;56:283-86.

[38] Levi M, Ten Cate H. Disseminated intravascular coagulation. N Engl J Med 1999; 341: 586–592.

[39] http://emedicine.medscape.com/article/126806-overview#a0199

[40] Huisse MG, Pease S, Hurtado-Nedelec M, et al: Leucocyte activation: The link between inflammation and coagulation during heatstroke. A study of patients during the 2003 heat wave in Paris. *Crit Care Med* 36:2288, 2008.

[41] Naumann RO & Weinstein L. Disseminated intravascular coagulation ± the clinician's dilemma. *Obstetrical and Gynecological Survey*1985; 40: 487-492.

[42] Glass JP (1993) The diagnosis and treatment of stroke in a patient with cancer: nonbacterial thrombotic endocarditis (NBTE): a case report and review. *Clin Neurol Neurosurg* 95: 315-318.

[43] Evans TR, Mansi JL, Bevan DH (1996) Trousseau's syndrome in association with ovarian carcinoma. *Cancer* 77: 2544-2549.

[44] Varki A. Trousseau's syndrome: multiple definitions and multiple mechanisms. Blo*od;2007 : 1723-1729.*

[45] Colman RW, Rubin RN: Disseminated intravascular coagulation due to malignancy. *Seminars in Oncology* 1990; 17: 172-186.

[46] Toh CH, Dennis M. Disseminated intravascular coagulation. *BMJ.* 2003 Oct 25:327:974-7.

In: Disseminated Intravascular Coagulation (DIC)   ISBN: 978-1-62948-323-8
Editor: Balwinder Singh   © 2014 Nova Science Publishers, Inc.

Chapter II

Risk Factors for Disseminated Intravascular Coagulation

Akhilesh Kumar Tiwari, MD[1], Rajiv Ratan Singh, MD[2],*
Rishi Raj Sanjay, MD[3], Naveen Ganjoo, MD[4]
and Balwinder Singh, MD[5]

[1] Department of Anaesthesia and Critical Care,
National University Hospial, Singapore
[2] Department of Anaesthesia, SGPGIMS, Lucknow, Uttar Pradesh, India
[3] Department of Anacsthesia, Batra Hospital and Research Centre,
New Delhi, India
[4] Department of Medical Gastroenterology,
BGS Global Hospital, Bangalore
[5] Division of Pulmonary and Critical Care Medicine,
Mayo Clinic, Rochester, Minnesota, US

Abstract

Disseminated intravascular coagulation [DIC] is an acquired
hypercoagulable syndrome, also known as consumption coagulopathy or

---

* Corresponding Author address: Dr. Akhilesh Kumar Tiwari, National University Hospial, 5
Lower Kent Ridge Road, Singapore. Email:draktiwari11@gmail.com.

defibrination syndrome. DIC is characterized by a systematic activation of coagulation cascade, contributing to the widespread intravascular fibrin generation and clot formation, resulting in inadequate blood supply to organs and leading to organ failure. DIC complicates an underlying illness, occurring in about 1% and 2% of hospital and ICU admissions respectively, and thus worsening their clinical outcomes. Despite appropriate management, patients with DIC have a high mortality ranging from 43%-78%. Thus, an early detection and rapid treatment of DIC will improve patient's outcome.

There is no established way of diagnosing DIC, and a number of laboratory and clinical indices were proposed by international experts for the diagnosis of DIC. The diagnosis of DIC is usually a combination of both clinical and laboratory parameters. In 1987, the Japanese Ministry of Health and Welfare proposed first proposed the criteria for diagnosis of DIC. After a decade, the Scientific Subcommittee on DIC of the International Society on Thrombosis and Hemostasis [ISTH] proposed a simple algorithm to diagnose DIC in 2001, into overt and non-overt DIC, which is followed largely over the last decade. After ISTH score, new criteria were proposed by the Japanese group known as the Japanese Association for Acute Medicine [JAAM] score. These scores were an attempt for the rapid detection of DIC, and improving patient outcomes.

The management of patients with DIC is primarily directed against the underlying etiology. However, in general patients who are bleeding or are considered being at higher risk of bleeding, with a platelet count of less than 50 X 10 9 / L are considered for platelet transfusion. Prophylactic transfusion of both platelets and fresh frozen plasma is not indicated in patients diagnosed to be suffering from DIC. Refractory and severe hypofibrinogenemia may be managed by fibrinogen concentrate and or cryoprecipitate. Heparin has also been used with variable success in patients with predominant thrombosis. Various other newer modalities such as antithrombin have been used with variable success and are currently the areas of research interest.

The present chapter will focus in details about the most important risk factors for DIC.

Introduction

Disseminated Intravascular Coagulation (DIC) is a potentially fatal syndrome, complicating various underlying disorders such as sepsis, malignancy, haematological disorders, trauma and obstetric conditions [1-3]. DIC is commonly encountered in the Intensive care setting and if not managed aggressively may rapidly lead to the development of multiple organ dysfunction syndromes [MODS]. MODS developing in patients with DIC can be either ischemic or inflammatory in origin [4]. DIC is a clinicopathologocal syndrome, characterized by a combination of thrombosis and hemorrhage, which is often fulminant and has been referred to as "Malignant Syndrome"[5]. Presence of DIC further complicates the management of the primary disorder and is associated with very high mortality and clinically significant morbidity.

The term DIC was coined by Hardway and McKay in the year 1959 [6] and since then various terminologies have been proposed like consumption coagulopathy, systemic intravascular fibrin formation, consumptive defibrination and systemic thrombohemorrhagic syndrome [7] although; DIC has been the most popular and widely adopted. This condition was reported for the first time in the year 1901 as "temporary hemophilia" in two parturients, one of whom had a retained dead fetus and the other suffered from placental abruption [8].

Following this several case reports were published, reporting the development of DIC in patients suffering from haematological malignancies and solid cancers [9]. There have been a number of diagnostic criteria proposed for the diagnosis of the DIC notable among them includes the criteria proposed by Japanese Ministry of Health and Welfare [JMHW], International Society on Thrombosis and Haemostasis [ISTH] and Japanese Association of Acute Care Medicine [JAAM] [10-12].

In the present chapter our focus will be directed towards the various risk factors of DIC.

Clinical Settings

One thing every clinician should have in mind is that this entity does not occur on its own, and is almost always associated with an underlying pathology which is associated with activation of coagulation system. There are various disorders associated with the pathogenesis of the DIC and are enumerated in table 1, and the important ones will be discussed further.

Table 1. Clinical conditions associated with the development of DIC [13-16]

Sepsis	<ul><li>Bacterial – Gram negative bacilli, Staphylococci, Streptococci, Meningococci</li><li>Viral – Herpes, rubella, smallpox, acute hepatitis, viral hemorrhagic fever, Arbovirus, Varicella, Variola, Rubella, Cytomegalovirus</li><li>Mycotic – Acute Histoplasmosis, Aspergillosis</li><li>Parasitic – Malaria, Kala-azar, Histoplasmosis.</li><li>Rickettsial - Rocky Mountain Spotted Fever.</li></ul>
Malignancy	<ul><li>Carcinomas (Prostrate, Pancreas, Ovary, Breast, Lung etc.)</li><li>Miscellaneous (Metastatic Carcinoid, Rhabdomyosarcoma, Neuroblastoma and others)</li><li>Cancer Chemotherapy</li><li>Tumour Lysis Syndrome</li></ul>
Obstetrical Disorders	<ul><li>Amniotic fluid embolism</li><li>Placental abruption</li><li>Retained fetus syndrome</li><li>Eclampsia</li><li>Abortion</li><li>Abdominal Pregnancy</li><li>Degenerating Hydatiform Mole</li><li>Intrauterine Fetal Death</li><li>HELLP* syndrome</li><li>Uterine atony</li><li>Bilateral renal cortical necrosis of pregnancy</li></ul>

Tissue Destruction and Trauma	<ul><li>Severe pancreatitis</li><li>Burns</li><li>Crush injuries and large massive trauma</li><li>Extensive Tissue necrosis</li><li>Rhabdomyolysis</li><li>Extensive Surgical Intervention</li><li>Fat Embolism</li></ul>
Toxic or Immunological Reactions	<ul><li>Snake bite</li><li>Recreational drug use (Cocaine)</li><li>Transfusion reaction</li><li>Minor hemolysis</li><li>Transplant rejection</li></ul>
Vascular abnormalities	<ul><li>Kasabach-Merritt syndrome</li><li>Large aneurysm</li><li>Giant Hemangiomas</li><li>Collagen Vascular Disorders</li><li>Autoimmune conditions – rheumatoid arthritis, systemic lupus erythematosus, Sjogren's syndrome, dermatomyositis, scleroderma etc.</li></ul>
Liver disorder	<ul><li>Obstructive jaundice.</li><li>Acute hepatic failure</li></ul>

Table 1. (Continued)

Hemopoietic Disorders	<ul><li>Acute Leukaemia's specially acute promyelocytic leukaemia</li><li>Intravascular hemolysis (Transfusion reaction, PNH, drug induced and sickle cell disease)</li><li>Histiocytic Medullary Reticulosis</li></ul>
Genetic Predisposition	<ul><li>Protein C deficiency</li><li>Protein S Deficiency</li><li>Decreased activity of Antithrombin inhibitory pathway</li><li>Factor V Leiden</li></ul>
Miscellaneous	<ul><li>Congestive Failure with Pulmonary emboli</li><li>Myocardial Infarction</li><li>Shock</li><li>Hypothermia</li><li>Cardiac arrest</li><li>Drowning especially in fresh water</li><li>Hemolytic uremic Syndrome</li><li>Acute Glomerulitis</li><li>Prosthetic Devices</li><li>Frost bite</li><li>Hyperthermia and Heat Stroke</li><li>Acidosis</li></ul>

Sepsis

DIC has been known to complicate up to 25-50% of sepsis cases [17-18], leading to MODS [19]. DIC associated with sepsis is usually not confined to one particular organism or type but may be seen complicating infections caused by bacteria, viruses and parasites as well. Among infectious organism it's the gram negative organism which has been traditionally associated with development of DIC. However, as opposed to the popular belief the incidence of clinically overt DIC in both gram negative and gram positive sepsis seems to be equal [13, 20]

Sepsis is a serious clinical entity and is one of the common causes of mortality in the non cardiac intensive care units [21]. Sepsis is almost always associated with underlying impairment of haemostasis which may range from isolated thrombocytopenia and sub clinical hypercoagulability to a full blown DIC [19]. It usually starts with intravascular activation of coagulation system followed by deposition of fibrin in the microvasculature and thus leading to the development of DIC which may progress further to MODS if not managed aggressively.

Main factors leading to the development of DIC are endotoxins [from gram negative bacteria] or exotoxin [e.g., staphylococcal alpha toxin]. These toxins results in activation of toll like receptors, which in turn stimulates nuclear factor kappa B. Hence severe systemic inflammation which accompanies sepsis is also associated with the release of various proinflammatory cytokines and complement activation which are thought to be the initial triggering factor [19].

The main hallmark of the coagulopathy in sepsis is the underlying imbalance between intravascular fibrin formation and its removal. Activation of coagulation and inhibition of fibrinolysis are mainly mediated by tumor necrosis factor [TNF] α, Interleukin [IL] 1 and IL-6 [18-20]. TNF α is also involved in the activation of coagulation cascade via IL-6. Endotoxemia also activates factor XII leading to the conversion of prekallikrein to kallikrein and kininogen into kinins which are responsible for increased vascular permeability, vasodilatation and shock [22].

Meningococcemia in addition is also associated with presence of microparticles derived from platelets and granulocytes which have been proposed to be possessing procoagulant activity [23]. So, the initiating factor is usually endo or exotoxin originating from the organism, with the most important mechanism being the activation of extrinsic pathway mediated by the interaction of tissue factor following endothelial damage. These bacterial endotoxins have also been associated with the activation of the intrinsic pathway mediated by factor XII [24].

Gram negative bacteria are one of the most common, but, not the only organisms responsible for the DIC in sepsis. Other agents such as gram positive bacteria [Staphylococcus aureus, Streptococcus pneumoniae, clostridium perferinges], viral infections such as hepatitis have also been occasionally associated with the occurrence of DIC. Table 1 shows an exhaustive list of infective pathogens linked with the occurrence of DIC. Bleeding in patients with DIC is usually triggered by the activation of coagulation system leading to the consumption of platelets and other coagulation factors. DIC in patients with sepsis can be caused due to the following mechanisms [19, 25].

a)   Procoagulant up regulation: Mediated primarily by the tissue factor which leads to increased thrombin production.
b)   Downregulation of physiological anticoagulation:
   a)   Decreased antithrombin.
   b)   Decreased protein C activity.
c)   Inadequate amount of tissue factor pathway inhibitor.
c)   Suppression of fibrinolysis
   a)   Mediated by the Plasminogen activator inhibitor 1 which are released by endothelial cells.
   b)   Thrombin activatable fibrinolysis inhibitor [TAFI] is also responsible for suppression of fibrinolysis.

Malignancy

Malignancy is considered to be the third most common cause of DIC only after sepsis and trauma with close to 7% of cases related to an underlying malignancy [24]. The commonest haematological manifestation associated with malignancy is bleeding secondary to thrombocytopenia arising as a result of chemotherapy, radiotherapy or due to bone marrow involvement [26]. But, DIC is also considered to be one of the important causes of bleeding in patient with malignant disorders. The first case of fatal hemorrhage in acute leukaemia was reported in the year 1935 [27]. About 60% of patients with malignancy may have thrombosis and variable degree of hypercoagulability.

Patients with metastatic tumour also tend to have increased platelet turnover with decreased life span. About ten to 15% of patients with metastatic tumour have DIC of variable degree and 15% of patients suffering from acute leukaemia may present with DIC [1].

Malignancy in itself is a hypercoagulable condition, with advancing age, male sex, presence of primary tumour necrosis and advanced stage further increasing the risk of developing DIC in the malignant disorders [28, 29]. Among the malignancies, the haematological malignancies are most often complicated by the DIC. Acute promyelocytic leukaemia [APL], a variant of acute leukemia, is associated with DIC in majority of the patients [30], and this causation has been related to the release of various pro-coagulant enzymes present in the abnormally large granules present in leukemic promyelocytes [30-33]. Surface of promyelocytic blast cells contains procoagulant which has action similar to thromboplastin and is capable of initiating the clotting mechanism. These cancer cells in APL have also been found to have a higher level of annexin II which leads to increased production of plasmin and hence the unopposed fibrinolysis may also lead to bleeding [34]. Among solid tumours, cancer of lung, breast, stomach, prostate, pancreas, ovary and bile tract are few of the common ones found to be associated with DIC [35-37].

The development of DIC in patients with malignancy is multifactorial and is not well understood but may involve the activation and release of various procoagulant factors. Release of tissue factor, activation of leucocytes coupled with direct activation of prothrombinase complex by mucin or specific cancer procoagulant are few of the mechanism described [38]. In addition of the above mechanisms, activation and aggregation of platelets, suppression of fibrinolysis cytokine mediated defective anticoagulation also plays a role in the activation of coagulation and ensuing the procoagulant state of malignant conditions as already discussed.

Other important factor which is responsible for maintaining hypercoagulability is the presence of a calcium dependent cysteine protease which has been found in malignant and fetal tissue. This is responsible for the direct activation of factor X, independent of the activity of tissue factor/ factor VIIa complex [39,40]. Another protease Hepsin normally found on the cell surface of hepatocytes and also on few tumour cells also initiates coagulation by independently activating factor VII [41]. These procoagulants have been associated with the activation of intrinsic coagulation pathway. Other forms of leukaemia have also been linked with DIC, although with a much lower frequency of up to 1-2 %. This is the reason why before initiating chemotherapy in these patients, DIC should be ruled out because the lysis of the leukemic cells as a result of chemotherapy may further worsen a sub acute DIC [30]. Other possible mechanism responsible for the DIC in haematological malignancy is profound immunosuppression and neutropenia arising as a result of various forms of therapies for the management of these haematological malignancies, predisposing the patient to various forms of infections like bacterial, viral, fungal or protozoal. These infections in there own right also predisposes an individual to a higher risk of DIC.

Various solid neoplasms have also been associated with occurrence of almost all the varieties of DIC like subclinical DIC, subacute DIC, chronic DIC and acute fulminant DIC. Different theories have been proposed explaining the likelihood of DIC in these patients. Patients with solid tumours express tissue factor on their cell surface which in combination with factor VII tends to activate intrinsic pathway of coagulation system. Pancreatic, breast and prostate cancer are one of the few solid malignancies commonly found to have association with DIC [26]. As discussed already these tumour cells also express cysteine protease which can activate factor X. In addition to these general features, various other types of solid organ malignancy precipitate DIC by virtue of certain typical features. DIC for example is the most common haematological disorder encountered in patients with prostate cancer. Prostate cancer may lead to DIC because of the release of certain thromboplastic substances into the blood stream. Pancreatic tumours release trypsin like substances which leads to the activation of factor X. Mucin like substances released by various gastrointestinal tumours have been implicated as a causative factor for DIC.

Extensive Tissue Damage

Tissue trauma can be a result of natural disaster or may develop as a result of road traffic accident, assault, burns or chemical injuries among various other causes. Road traffic accident is one of the leading causes of death and morbidity world over. DIC complicating a case of trauma is usually responsible for late morbidity. Trauma patients with systemic inflammatory response syndrome [SIRS] are at higher risk, with more than 50 % of these patients developing DIC [24, 42- 43]. Trauma patients with head injury and extensive transfusion are also at increased risk of developing DIC. The evidence relating head injury and consumption coagulopathy started emerging in the year 1974, when Goodnight et al. [44] and Strinchini et al. [45] in two different studies demonstrated defibrination in cases of head injury. Drayer and colleague in the following year described a case of DIC in a patient with head injury [46]. Coagulopathy after head injury is most prevalent in the first 24 hours, and is more commonly encountered in females. The risk of developing coagulopathy increases with worsening Glasgow coma score [GCS] as the level of fibrin degradation products have been positively linked with the degree of brain damage [47].

Patients with extensive trauma are prone to develop early coagulopathy [48]; rather it's not wrong to consider a patient with trauma to be having some sort of coagulopathy on admission. This coagulopathy causes bleeding from various sites like mucosal surface and serosal surface and also from various vascular access site in addition to the bleeding from wound and surgical site.

There are two phases of coagulopathy encountered in these patients: an early phase of bleeding and a late phase of thrombosis [47]. Coagulopathy arising in patients with trauma is multifactorial and is still not well understood. Release of various tissue enzymes, phospholipids and fat from injured and damaged tissue leading to the release and activation of a host of cytokines has been blamed for DIC in patients with extensive tissue injury. The high levels of these inflammatory cytokines lead to the activation of tissue factor and subsequent coagulation pathway. Widespread activation of coagulation leads to the consumption coagulopathy which is a common finding in trauma patients.

To simplify, in patients with trauma we have two mechanisms contributing to the pathogenesis: the release of various procoagulant factors coupled with the systemic inflammatory response syndrome both of which are involved in activation and expression of tissue factor on monocytes and various other cells. These contributing factors are further aggravated by the decreased endogenous fibrinolytic activity.

Other non traumatic causes of tissue destruction include burns, extensive surgery and inflammatory conditions like pancreatitis. Anemia, coagulopathy, leukocytosis and thrombocytopenia have been reported with variable degree in pancreatitis [49]. This condition predominantly involves microcirculation leading to the release various inflammatory tissue mediators and endothelial damage. Exact pathogenesis of DIC in these patients is still open to investigators, but the blood picture consistent with DIC has been reported in patients suffering from DIC. However, role of pancreatic enzymes and vascular injury has been proposed as the likely cause. These patients have increased tendency to develop thrombosis both deep vein thrombosis and microthrombi [50-52]. Another potential cause of DIC arising as a result of extensive tissue trauma which deserves mention here is burn. Burn injury results in the entry of cellular debris and necrotic tissue in the bloodstream. This debris usually has strong thromboplastic activity mainly because of expression and release of tissue factor which results in the explosive production of thrombin ultimately leading to DIC. Other factor which may also play a supporting role in the pathogenesis is the possible immunological and inflammatory injury to the bodily tissue leading to the release of various inflammatory mediators and cytokines [53].

DIC in Obstetric Practice

There are number of obstetric conditions which predispose a parturient to increased risk of DIC. Pregnancy in itself, due to various physiological changes is a hypercoagulable state predisposing women to varying severity of DIC ranging from a less severe thrombotic form to a full blown one. The incidence of DIC with in the obstetric population is extremely variable depending upon the suspected underlying cause. Before discussing further, it's apt at this juncture to discuss the physiological changes which make a parturient hypercoagulable and therefore prone to DIC. Most of these changes are usually hormone driven. During pregnancy, there is significant increase in the plasma concentration of coagulation factors mainly VII, VIII, IX, X and XII which usually returns back to normal after delivery [54]. This is also accompanied by significant increase in the concentration of certain procoagulant factors like fibrinogen along with suppression of fibrinolysis. [55-57]. Placenta has also been proposed as one of the contributing factor in the pathogenesis of DIC [57, 58]. Phospholipids and tissue factor released by placenta during pregnancy further stimulate the release and activation of factor VII. Trophoblastic lining of placenta has also been implicated in the production of various haemostatic regulators like thrombomodulin, protein C receptor and tissue factor and these changes result in subsequent fibrin deposition [59]. These Trophoblastic cells have also been implicated in the production of endothelial protein C receptor and tissue factor pathway inhibitor [60-61]. Pregnancy is also associated with disturbance in the endogenous fibrinolytic activity to a variable degree [58].

Table 2. Obstetric causes of DIC

Amniotic Fluid Embolism [64-65]	1. 1in 8000 to 1 in 30,000 births. 2. Associated with maternal mortality of 60-80%. 3. Occurs due to entry of Amniotic fluid into the maternal circulation and subsequently in the pulmonary vasculature leading to circulatory collapse. 4. Amniotic fluid contains high concentration of plasminogen pro-activators. It activates factor X in the presence of calcium and also inhibits fibrinolytic system. 5. The manifestation of the syndrome does not depend on the amount of the fluid entering into the circulation, and hence anaphylactic component has also been proposed as the likely cause.
Abruptio Placenta [58, 64, 66]	1. There is about 10% risk of developing DIC in these patients. 2. Release of placental enzymes, tissue thromboplastin and various procoagulants into the uterus and subsequently into the maternal circulation has been implicated as the likely cause of DIC in this subgroup.
Intrauterine Fetal death [64]	1. Incidence of developing DIC in these patients have been reported to be as high as 50% if the dead fetus has been retained for upto 5 weeks. 2. This condition is usually associated with subacute or chronic DIC, that progress into more severe fulminant form if therapeutic measures are not put in place. 3. Various tissue enzymes and procoagulant released from the necrosed fetal tissue has been implicated behind the pathogenesis of DIC in cases of intrauterine fetal death.

Table 2. (Continued)

Pre-eclampsia, Eclampsia	1. Eclampsia and preeclampsia is one of the commonest obstetric condition associated with coagulopathy. 2. Pre-eclampsia occurs due to abnormal maternal response to placentation, the extent of which usually determined the severity of the disease. 3. Thrombocytopenia is considered to be an early indicator of possible DIC in this high risk group and arises mainly due to its increased consumption.
HELLP Syndrome [58, 64, 67]	1. It's considered to be an advanced stage of Eclampsia preeclampsia and forms one end of this spectrum. It has an incidence of 0.17%-0.85% of all live birth. 2. A combination of factors like endothelial dysfunction, inflammatory mediators and the activation of platelets and cytokines predispose these patients to develop DIC.
Abortion [64, 68-71]	1. Haematological changes similar to DIC have been demonstrated in patients where abortion was induced by hypertonic solution of saline and urea. 2. Saline induced abortion is usually associated with subclinical DIC; however, 1 in 400 to 1 in 1000 cases may be associated with severe form of DIC. 3. Likely cause behind the development of DIC in these patients has been proposed to be the release of tissue thromboplastin into the maternal circulation.
Acute Fatty liver of pregnancy [72-74]	1. It was described in 1934 as "yellow acute atrophy of the liver" and in 1940 was described as a specific entity. 2. It has an incidence of 1 in 13000 deliveries, and is associated with DIC. 3. Severe Hepatic dysfunction has been proposed as the most likely cause of DIC in this subgroup of patients [75].

Hemodilution observed in pregnant patients coupled with increased platelet destruction with resultant thrombocytopenia has also been suggested to play a role. As the duration of pregnancy increases the concentration of factor VIII and von Willebrand factor antigen also increases and concentration of protein C and S progressively decreases.

Overall incidence of DIC in obstetric practice has been estimated to be about 1 in 1355 deliveries [62]. The first report linking amniotic fluid embolism with DIC was provided by Steiner and Lushbaugh in 1941 [63-64]. Association of DIC with amniotic fluid embolism is one of the catastrophic complications seen in obstetric practice. The following table enumerates the important obstetric causes of DIC with their salient points.

Genetic Risk Factors

Occasional cases of DIC have been reported to occur spontaneously without an underlying disease. A genetic defect involving any of the factors taking part in coagulation cascade or fibrinolytic pathway may predispose an individual to increased risk of developing DIC. One such example is the occurrence of neonatal purpura fulminans in children suffering from protein C or protein S deficiency. Individuals who are heterozygotes for these deficiencies have been traditionally considered to be at high risk of developing DIC without an underlying disorder. Cases linking these defects with DIC and neonatal purpura fulminans have are well documented in the literature [76-78].

Protein C is a glycoprotein which circulates in plasma in an inactive form. It's a vitamin K dependent factor which also requires the presence of protein S and anionic phospholipids for its activity [77]. Protein C gets converted into its active form [APC] by the action of thrombin-thrombomodulin complex. APC is a naturally occurring anticoagulant which degrades the activated factor V and VIII, thereby decreasing the procoagulant activity [79, 80]. Protein C deficiency is an autosomal dominant condition which may present clinically with symptoms of variable severity ranging from purpura fulminans to venous thromboembolism and DIC [77]. Incidence of protein C deficiency is highly variable and is about 1 in 300 for heterozygous protein C deficiency [81], and 1 in 5,00,000 − 750,000 births for homozygous protein C deficiency [82].

Protein S is also vitamin K dependent glycoprotein, which is involved in the inactivation of factor Va, VIIa and Xa. It has been found to be circulating in both free and combined form and it's the free form which has been associated with anticoagulant activity. Incidence of protein S deficiency is variable and affects about 1 in 700 healthy individual, and the incidence of protein S deficiency increases to 3-6% in patients suffering from recurrent thrombosis or with family history of thrombosis [83]

Deficiency of both protein C and protein S has been associated with DIC [84 - 91]

Individual with genetic defect in the fibrinolytic pathway are also at increased risk of developing DIC. Other possible genetic causes which may increase the chances of DIC in a genetically susceptible individual are enumerated in table 3 [85].

Table 3. Genetic factors predisposing an individual to DIC

1) Protein C deficiency.
2) Protein S deficiency.
3) Factor V Leiden mutation.
4) Genetic alteration of proteins involved in fibrinolytic and anti-fibrinolytic pathway.
5) Genetically determined increased levels of procoagulants.

Vascular

Giant hemangiomas and large aortic aneurysm are associated with localised activation of coagulation cascade. Kasabach Merritt syndrome is one such condition where giant cavernous hemangioma. About 25% cases of giant cavernous hemangioma may be associated with low grade DIC; whereas, about 50% of patient with hereditary hemorrhagic telangiectasia may have low grade DIC. The probable reason behind the development of DIC in these patients has been linked to endothelial damage and stasis of the blood in these large vascular malformations. Aortic aneurysms however are a rarer cause of DIC, with only 0.5-0.6% of cases occurring because of it [92-94]

It has also been observed in about 3-4 % of patients with large abdominal aortic aneurysm. Other vascular conditions like Raynaud's syndrome, diabetic angiopathy, and autoimmune disorder may also develop compensated DIC [64].

Cardiovascular Conditions

Various cardiovascular conditions have been associated with the development of low grade subacute DIC. Patients suffering from acute myocardial infarction have also been reported to suffer from DIC [64]. Exact mechanism underlying the pathogenesis of DIC in cardiovascular disorder is not very well understood but a combination of factor including shock; hypoxia, acidosis and stasis have been suggested. Infarcted myocardial tissue has also been shown to release thromboplastin.

Prosthetic Devices [64]

Presence of various prosthetic devices in the body has been known to be a triggering factor behind the development of DIC. Intra aortic balloon pump and Le Veen or Denver shunt have been known to precipitate DIC. Insertion of these devices is associated with release and activation of various procoagulants, consumption coagulopathy and generation of microthrombi. Occurrence of DIC in peritoneovenus shunt primarily occurs because of entry of endotoxins and procoagulants into the blood stream from the ascitic fluid. It has been said that the occurrence of DIC in these cases can be decreased by draining the ascitic fluid

Toxic Reactions

Snake bite [especially Crotalidae i.e., pit vipers] and bee sting have been reported to be associated with DIC.. Snake venom has action similar to thrombin and tends to form fibrin [95-96].Unlike stable fibrin molecules, this unstable fibrin polymer is vulnerable to fibrinolyis and phagocytosis by reticuloendothelial system. This imparts the property of inducing various types of coagulopathy to snake venom ranging from a simple thrombocytopenia to a full blown DIC. The prevalence of coagulopathy due to snake bites has been proposed to be between 36-50% [97]. Type of snake bite, site and time length of the bite have also been proposed to influence the development of the DIC in the patients.

Fatal cases of intravascular coagulation have been reported following anaphylactic shock after bee sting acupuncture [98]. DIC after bee stings is a rare complication; however, phospholipase A2 present in bee venom has been know to casue coagulation abnormalities [99-100].

Recreational use of cocaine has been linked to DIC and deserves its mention here. The exact pathogenesis is not well understood. Severe thrombocytopenia has been reported in individuals using cocaine by both intravenous and inhalational route. Exact mechanism behind this phenomenon is not well understood [101-102].

Thus, despite the recent evidnce of decrease in the incidence of DIC over the past decade, the mortality rate remains very high [103-104]. Thus, there is a need to identify risk factors of DIC early and manage appropriately to reduce the morbidity and mortality, and improve the outcomes [105].

In conclusion, this chapter provides an exhaustive review of various etiological factors responsible for DIC. The most common causes leading to the development of DIC are sepsis, trauma and maignancy. A high index of suspicion is usually required in these high risk cases to make an early diagnosis and initiate rapid and aggressive treatment to decrease mortality.

References

[1]   Levi M, Ten Cate H. Disseminated intravascular coagulation. *N Engl J Med* 1999; 341:586-592,

[2]   Muller-Berghaus G, ten Cate H, Levi M. Disseminated intravascular coagulation: clinical spectrum and established as well as new diagnostic approaches. *Thromb Haemost* 1999;82:706–12.

[3]   Levi M, de Jonge E, van der Poll T, ten Cate H. Advances in the understanding of the pathogenetic pathways of disseminated intravascular coagulation result in more insight in the clinical picture and better management strategies. *Semin Thromb Hemost* 2001; 27:569–75.

[4]   Levi M. Disseminated intravascular coagulation. *Crit Care Med* 2007;35:2191–5.

[5]   Ph. Cauchie, Ch. Cauchie, K. Zouaoui Boudjeltia, E. Carlier, N. Deschepper, D. Govaerts, M. Migaud-Fressart, B. Woodhams, and D. Brohe'e. Diagnosis and prognosis of overt disseminated intravascular coagulation in a general hospital – Meaning of the ISTH score system, Fibrin monomers, and Lipoprotein- C – Reactive Protein Complex formation *American Journal of Hematology* 81:414–419 2006.

[6] Ghazi A, Siddiq NM, Ali T, Jabbar S, Muhammad ZW. Deranged coagulation profile among obstetric patients. 2008; 24:135-137.

[7] Levi M, de Jonge E, van der Poll T. Sepsis and disseminated intravascular coagulation. *J Thromb Thrombolysis*. 2003; 16: 43-7.

[8] DeLee, JB A case of fatal hemorrhagic diathesis, with premature detachment of the placenta *Am J Obstet Dis Women Child*. 1901; 44:785

[9] H. Wada. Disseminated Intravascular coagulation. *Clinica Chimica Acta*.2004; 344:13-21.

[10] Takemitsu T, Wada H, Hatada T, Ohmori Y, Ishikura K, Takeda T, Sugiyama T, Yamada N, Maruyama K, Katayama N, Isaji S, Shimpo H, Kusunoki M, Nobori T. Prospective evaluation of three different diagnostic criteria for disseminated intravascular coagulation. *Thromb Haemost*. 2011;105:40-4.

[11] Taylor FB Jr, Toh CH, Hoots WK, Wada H, Levi M; Scientific Subcommittee on Disseminated Intravascular Coagulation [DIC] of the International Society on Thrombosis and Haemostasis [ISTH]. Towards definition, clinical and laboratory criteria, and a scoring system for disseminated intravascular coagulation. *Thromb Haemost*. 2001;86:1327-30.

[12] Gando S, Iba T, Eguchi Y, Ohtomo Y, Okamoto K, Koseki K, Mayumi T, Murata A, Ikeda T, Ishikura H, Ueyama M, Ogura H, Kushimoto S, Saitoh D, Endo S, Shimazaki S; Japanese Association for Acute Medicine Disseminated Intravascular Coagulation [JAAM DIC] Study Group. A multicenter, prospective validation of disseminated intravascular coagulation diagnostic criteria for critically ill patients: comparing current criteria. *Crit Care Med*. 2006;34:625-31.

[13] Dalainas I. Pathogenesis, diagnosis, and management of disseminated intravascular coagulation: a literature review. *Eur Rev Med Pharmacol Sci*. 2008;12:19-31.

[14] Naz H, Fawad A, Islam A, Shahid H, Abbasi AU. Disseminated intravascular coagulation. J Ayub Med Coll Abbottabad. 2011;23:111-3.

[15] http://www.ncbi.nlm.nih.gov/books/NBK6069/ accessed on 13 April 2013

[16] Bakshi S, Arya LS. Etiopathophysiology of disseminated intravascular coagulation. *J Assoc Physicians India*. 2003 Aug;51:796-800.

[17] Dempfle CE, Wurst M, Smolinski M, et al. Use of soluble fibrin antigen instead of D-dimer as fibrin-related marker may enhance the prognostic power of the ISTH overt DIC score. *Thromb Haemost* 2004; 91:812–818

[18] Dhainaut JF, Yan SB, Joyce DE, et al. Treatment effects of drotrecogin alfa [activated] in patients with severe sepsis with or without overt disseminated intravascular coagulation. *J Thromb Haemost* 2004; 2:1924–1933.

[19] Semeraro N, Ammollo CT, Semeraro F, Colucci M. Sepsis-associated disseminated intravascular coagulation and thromboembolic disease. *Mediterr J Hematol Infect Dis.* 2010 Aug 13;2[3]:e2010024. doi: 10.4084/MJHID.2010.024.

[20] Bone RC. Gram-positive organisms and sepsis.*Arch Intern Med* 1994; 154: 26-34.

[21] Zeerleder S, Hack CE, Wuillemin WA. Disseminated intravascular coagulation in sepsis. *Chest.* 2005 Oct: 128[4]:2864-75.

[22] Colman RW. Contact systems in infectious disease. *Rev Infect Dis* 1989; 11 Suppl 4:S689.

[23] Nieuwland R, Berckmans RJ, McGregor S, Böing AN, Romijn FP, Westendorp RG, Hack CE, Sturk A. Cellular origin and procoagulant properties of microparticles in meningococcal sepsis. *Blood.* 2000 Feb 1;95[3]:930-5.

[24] http://www.uptodate.com/contents/pathogenesis-and-etiology-of-disseminated-intravascular-coagulation accessed on 7 May 2013.

[25] Franchini M, Lippi G, Manzato F. Recent acquisitions in the pathophysiology, diagnosis and treatment of disseminated intravascular coagulation. *Thromb J.* 2006 Feb 21;4:4.

[26] Bick RL Coagulation abnormalities in malignancy: a review. *Semin Thromb Hemost.* 1992;18[4]:353-72.

[27] Sarris AH, Kempin S, Berman E, Michaeli J, Little C, Andreeff M, Gee T, Straus D, Gansbacher B, Filippa D, et al. High incidence of disseminated intravascular coagulation during remission induction of adult patients with acute lymphoblastic leukemia. *Blood.* 1992 Mar 1;79[5]:1305-10.

[28] Duran I, Tannock IF. Disseminated intravascular coagulation as the presenting sign of metastatic prostate cancer. *J Gen Intern Med.* 2006;21[11]:1206.

[29] Sallah S, Wan JY, Nguyen NP, Hanrahan LR, Sigounas G. Disseminated intravascular coagulation in solid tumors: clinical and pathologic study. *Thromb Haemost.* 2001;86:828–33.

[30] Colman RW, Rubin RN. Disseminated intravascular coagulation due to malignancy. *Semin Oncol.* 1990 Apr;17[2]:172-86.

[31] Sakurgawa N, Takahashi K, Hoshiyama M, JImbo C, Matsuoka M. Pathological cells as procoagulant substance of disseminated intravascular coagulation syndrome in acute promyelocytic syndrome. *Thromb Res.* 1976 Mar;8[3]:263-273.

[32] Savage RA, Hoffman GC, Lucas FV Jr. Morphology and cytochemistry of "microgranular" acute promyelocytic leukemia. *Am J Clin Pathol.* 1981 Apr;75[4]:548-52.

[33] Bauer KA, Rosenberg RD. Thrombin generation in acute promyelocytic leukemia. *Blood.* 1984 Oct;64[4]:791-6.

[34] Menell JS, Cesarman GM, Jacovina AT, et al. Annexin II and bleeding in acute promyelocytic leukemia [see comments]. *N Engl J Med.* 1999;340:994.

[35] Ludwig J, Kentos A, Creiner I, et al. Disseminated intravascular coagulation syndrome as manifestation of breast adenocarcinoma metastasis. *Rev Med Brux.* 1997;18:385-388.

[36] Ohtake N, Kurita S, Fukabor Y, et al. Clinical study on prostate cancer initially presenting with disseminated intravascular coagulation syndrome. Hinyokika Kiyo. 1998;44:387-390.

[37] Gouin-Thibault I, Achkar A, Samama MM. The thrombophilic state in cancer patients. *Acta Haematol.* 2001;106:33-42.

[38] A. Ravikumar, Vivek Sasindran, K. Senthil, John Samuel, Thirumaran. Disseminated Intravascular Coagulation syndrome — ENT surgeon's perspective. ndian *J Otolaryngol Head Neck Surg.* 2006 October; 58[4]: 384–386.

[39] Gordon SG, Miclicki WP. Cancer procoagulant: a factor X activator, tumor marker and growth factor from malignant tissue. *Blood Coagul Fibrinolysis* 1997; 8:73.

[40] Gordon SG, Franks JJ, Lewis B. Cancer procoagulant A: a factor X activating procoagulant from malignant tissue. *Thromb Res* 1975; 6:127.

[41] Kazama Y, Hamamoto T, Foster DC, Kisiel W: Hepsin, a putative membrane-associated serine protease, activates human factor VII and initiates a pathway of blood coagulation on the cell surface leading to thrombin formation. *J Biol Chem* 1995, 270:66-72.

[42] Gando S, Kameue T, Nanzaki S, Nakanishi Y. Disseminated intravascular coagulation is a frequent complication of systemic inflammatory response syndrome. *Thromb Haemost* 1996; 75:224.

[43] Gando S, Nanzaki S, Kemmotsu O. Disseminated intravascular coagulation and sustained systemic inflammatory response syndrome

predict organ dysfunctions after trauma: application of clinical decision analysis. *Ann Surg* 1999; 229:121.

[44] Goodnight SH, Kenoyer G, Rapaport SI, Patch MJ, Lee JA, Kurze T. Defibrination after brain-tissue destruction: A serious complication of head injury. *N Engl J Med.* 1974 May 9;290[19]:1043-7.

[45] Strinchini A, Baudo F, Nosari AM, Panzacchi G, de Cataldo F. Letter: Defibrination and head injury. *Lancet.* 1974 Oct 19; 2[7886]:957.

[46] Drayer BP, Poser CM. Disseminated intravascular coagulation and head trauma. Two case studies. *JAMA.* 1975 Jan 13;231[2]:174-5.

[47] Lippi G, Cervellin G. Disseminated intravascular coagulation in trauma injuries. *Semin Thromb Hemost.* 2010 Jun;36[4]:378-87.

[48] Tieu BH, Holcomb JB, Schreiber MA. Coagulopathy: its pathophysiology and treatment in the injured patient. *World J Surg.* 2007 May;31[5]:1055-64.

[49] Saif MW. DIC secondary to acute pancreatitis. *Clin Lab Haematol.* 2005 Aug;27[4]:274-82.

[50] Greipp PR, Brown JA, Gralnick HR. Defibrination in acute pancreatitis. *Ann Intern Med.* 1972 Jan;76[1]:73-6.

[51] Shinowara, G. Y., Sbutman, L. J., Welters, M. I., Ruth, M. E. and Walker, E. J.: Hypercoagulability in acute pancreatitis. *Amer. J. Surg.,* 105: 714-719, 1963.

[52] Agarwal M B, Kamdar M S, Bapat R D, Mehta B C, Rao S S, Rao P N. Consumptive coagulopathy and fibrinolysis in experimental acute pancreatitis. *J Postgrad Med* 1982;28:214]

[53] Lippi G, Ippolito L, Cervellin G. Disseminated intravascular coagulation in burn injury. *Semin Thromb Hemost.* 2010 Jun;36[4]:429-36.

[54] Bremme KA. Haemostatic changes in pregnancy. *Best Pract Res Clin Haematol* 2003;16[2]:153-168.

[55] Forbes CD & Greer IA. Physiology of haemostasis and the e€ect of pregnancy. In Greer IA, Turpie AGG & Forbes CD [eds] Haemostasis and Thrombosis in Obstetrics and Gynaecology, pp 1±25. London: Chapman & Hall, 1992.

[56] Stirling Y,Woolf L, North WR et al. Haemostasis in normal pregnancy. *Thrombosis and Haemostasis* 1984; 52: 176±182.

[57] Letsky EA. Disseminated Intravascular coagulation. *Best Practice & Research Clinical Obstetrics and Gynaecology* Vol. 15, No. 4, pp. 623-644, 2001.

[58] Disseminated Intravascular coagulation in Obstetric and Gynecological disorder. Martina Montagnana.

[59] Delorme MA, Burrows RF, Ofosu FA, Andrew M. Thrombin regulation in mother and fetus during pregnancy. *Semin Throm Hemost* 1992;18[1]:81-90.

[60] Maruyama I, Bell CE, Majerus PW. Thrombomodulin is found on endothelial of arteries, veins, capillaries ad lymphatics, and on syncytiotrophoblast of human placenta. *J Cell Biol* 1985;101[2]:363-371.

[61] Edstrom CS, Calhoun DA, Christensen RD. Expression of tissue factor pathway inhibitor in human fetal and placental tissue. *Early Hum Dev* 2000;59[2]:77-84.

[62] Tang BH. The critical analysis on diagnosis of disseminated intravascular coagulation with screening tests--a scoring system and related literature review. *J Ayub Med Coll Abbottabad.* 2007 Oct-Dec;19[4]:112-20.

[63] Steiner PE, Lushbough CC. Maternal pulmonary embolism by amniotic fluid as a cause of shock and unexplained deaths in obstetrics. *JAMA* 1941;117:1245.

[64] R L Bick. Disseminated Intravascular Coagulation: A review of Etiology, Pathophysiology, Diagnosis and Management: Guidelines for Care. *Clin Appl Thrombosis/Hemostasis* 8:1-31,2002.

[65] Clark SL, Montz FJ, Phelan JP. Hemodynamic alterations associated with amniotic fluid embolism: a reappraisal. *Am J Obstet Gynecol* 1985; 151: 617-21.

[66] Sher G. Pathogenesis and management of uterineinertia complicating abruption placentae with consumptive coagulopathy. *Am. J. Obstet Gynecol* 1977; 129: 164-70.

[67] Jecko Thachil , Cheng-Hock Toh. Disseminated intravascular coagulation in obstetric disorders and its acute haematological management. *Blood Reviews* 23 [2009] 167–176.

[68] Grundy MFB & Craven ER. Consumption coagulopathy after intra-amniotic urea. *British Medical Journal* 1976; 2: 677±678.

[69] Mackenzie IZ, Sayers L, Bonnar J et al. Coagulation changes during second trimester abortion induced by intra-amniotic prostaglandin E2‡ and hypertonic solutions. *Lancet* 1975; ii: 1066±1069.

[70] Spivak JL, Spangler DB & Bell WR. Defibrinogenation after intraamniotic injection of hypertonic saline. *New England Journal of Medicine* 1972; 287: 321±323.

[71]   Stander RW, Flessa HC & Glueck HI Changes in maternal coagulation factors after intraamniotic injection of hypertonic saline. *Obstetrics and Gynecology* 1971; 37: 660±666.

[72]   Stander HJ, Cadden JF. Acute yellow atrophy of the liver in pregnancy. *Am J Obstet Gynecol* 1934; 28: 61-69

[73]   Sheehan HL. The pathology of acute yellow atrophy and delayed chloroform poisoning. *J Obstet Gyneco Br Emp* 1940; 47: 49-62.

[74]   Ibdah JA. Acute fatty liver of pregnancy: an update on pathogenesis and clinical implications. *World J Gastroenterol* 2006 Dec 14:12[46]:7397-404.

[75]   Nihal Al Riyami, Abdullan Al-Harthy, Fehmida Zia. Atypical case of acute fatty liver of pregnancy. Sultan Qaboos Univ Med J. 2011 November;11[4]:507-510.

[76]   Goldenberg NA, Manco-Johnson MJ. Protein C deficiency. *Haemophilia.* 2008 Nov;14[6]:1214-21.

[77]   Tiwari AK, Tomar GS, Tayal S, Chadha M, Kapoor M. Anaesthetic significance and management of a child with neonatal purpura fulminans. *Indian J Anaesth.* 2012 May-Jun; 56[3]: 283–286.

[78]   Dahlbäck B. Advances in understanding pathogenic mechanisms of thrombophilic disorders. Blood. 2008 Jul 1;112[1]:19-27. doi: 10.1182/blood-2008-01-077909.

[79]   Suzuki K, Stenflo J, Dahlback B, Teodorsson B. Inactivation of human coagulation factor V by activated protein C. *J Biol Chem.* 1983;258:1914–1920.

[80]   Fulcher CA, Gardiner JE, Griffin JH, Zimmerman TS. Proteolytic inactivation of human factor VIII procoagulant protein by activated human protein C and its analogy with factor V. *Blood.* 1984;63:486–489.

[81]   Miletich J, Sherman L, Broze G Jr. Absence of thrombosis in subjects with heterozygous protein C deficiency. *N Engl J Med.* 1987;317:991–996.

[82]   Marlar RA, Mastovich S. Hereditary protein C deficiency: a review of the genetics, clinical presentation, diagnosis and treatment. *Blood Coagul Fibrinolysis.* 1990; 1:319–330

[83]   Marlar RA, Mastovich S. Hereditary protein C deficiency: a review of the genetics, clinical presentation, diagnosis and treatment. *Blood Coagul Fibrinolysis.* 1990; 1:319–330.

[84]   http://emedicine.medscape.com/article/205582-overview#a0199 accessed on 7th May 2013.

[85] http://www.ncbi.nlm.nih.gov/books/NBK6069/ accessed on 6th May 2013.

[86] Gerson WT, Dickerman JD, Bovill EG, Golden E. Severe acquired protein C deficiency in purpura fulminans associated with disseminated intravascular coagulation: treatment with protein C concentrate. *Pediatrics*. 1993;91:418–422.

[87] Powars D, Larsen R, Johnson J, Hulbert T, Sun T, Patch MJ, Francis R, Chan L. Epidemic meningococcemia and purpura fulminans with induced protein C deficiency. *Clin Infect Dis*. 1993;17:254– 261.

[88] Griffin JH, Mosher DF, Zimmerman TS, Kleiss AJ. Protein C, an antithrombotic protein, is reduced in hospitalized patients with intravascular coagulation. *Blood*. 1982;60:261–264.

[89] Fourrier F, Chopin C, Goudemand J, Hendrycx S, Caron C, Rime A, Marey A, Lestavel P. Septic shock, multiple organ failure, and disseminated intravascular coagulation. Compared patterns of antithrombin III, protein C, and protein S deficiencies [see comments] *Chest*. 1992;101:816–823.

[90] Alessi MC, Aillaud MF, BoyerNeumann C, Viard L, Camboulives J, JuhanVague I. Cutaneous necrosis associated with acquired severe protein S deficiency *Thromb Haemost*. 1993;69:524–526.

[91] Zenz W, Muntean W. Cutaneous necrosis associated with acquired severe protein S deficiency *Thromb Haemost*. 1994;71:396.

[92] Falanga A, Rickles FR. Management of thrombohemorrhagic syndromes in hematologic malignancies. *Hematology* 2007;165- 171.

[93] Siebert WT, Natelson EA. Chronic consumption coagulopathy accompanying abdominal aortic aneurysm. *Arch Surg* 1976;111:539-541.

[94] Aboulafia DM, Aboulafia ED. Aortic aneurysm-induced disseminated intravascular coagulation. *Ann Vasc Surg* 1996;10:396-405..

[95] Retzios AD, Markland FS., Jr Purification, characterization, and fibrinogen cleavage sites of three fibrinolytic enzymes from the venom of Crotalus basiliscus basiliscus. *Biochemistry*. 1992;31:4547–4557.

[96] Retzios AD, Markland FS. Fibrinolytic enzymes from the venoms of Agkistrodon contortrix contortrix and Crotalus basiliscus basiliscus: cleavage site specificity towards the alpha-chain of fibrin. *Thromb Res*. 1994;74:355–367

[97] Singletary EM, Rochman AS, Bodmer JC, Holstege CP. Envenomation. *Med Clin North Am*.2005;89:1195–1224.

[98] Jae Woo Jung, Eun Ju Jeon, Jeong Wook Kim, Jae Chol Choi, Jong Wook Shin, Jae Yeol Kim, In Won Park,and Byoung Whui Choi. A fatal case of Intravascular coagulation after Bee sting acupuncture. *Allergy Asthma Immunol Res.* 2012 March; 4[2]: 107–109.

[99] Petroianu G, Liu J, Helfrich U, Maleck W, Rüfer R. Phospholipase A2-induced coagulation abnormalities after bee sting. *Am J Emerg Med.* 2000;18:22–27.

[100] França FO, Benvenuti LA, Fan HW, Dos Santos DR, Hain SH, Picchi-Martins FR, Cardoso JL, Kamiguti AS, Theakston RD, Warrell DA. Severe and fatal mass attacks by 'killer' bees [Africanized honey bees--Apis mellifera scutellata] in Brazil: clinicopathological studies with measurement of serum venom concentrations. *Q J Med.* 1994;87:269–282.

[101] Roth D, Alarcon FJ, Fernandez JA, et al: Acute rhabdomyolysis associated with cocaine intoxication. *N Engl J Med* 1988; 319:673-677.

[102] Leissinger CA: Severe thrombocytopenia associated with cocaine use. *Ann Intern Med* 1990; 112:708-710.

[103] Singh B, Hanson AC, Alhurani R, Wang S, Herasevich V, Cartin-Ceba R, Kor DJ, Gangat N, Li Gl. Trends in the incidence and outcomes of disseminated intravascular coagulation in critically ill patients (2004-2010): A population-based study. *Chest.* 2013;143:1235-42.

[104] Singh B, Gajic O, Li G. Incidence And Outcome Of Disseminated Intravascular Coagulation (DIC) In Olmsted County, Minnesota (2004-2010)-A Population Based Cohort Study. *Am J Respir Crit Care Med.* 2012;185:A6063.

[105] Singh B, Ahmed A, Alhurani R, Hanson A, Franco P, Gajic O, Li G. Outcome of Critically ill Patients With Disseminating Intravascular Coagulation: A Population-Based Study. *Chest.* 2012;142:304A.

In: Disseminated Intravascular Coagulation (DIC)   ISBN: 978-1-62948-323-8
Editor: Balwinder Singh   © 2014 Nova Science Publishers, Inc.

Chapter III

Thrombomodulin and Disseminated Intravascular Coagulation

Shu-Min Lin MD and Han-Pin Kuo MD, PhD*
Department of Thoracic Medicine, Chang Gung Memorial Hospital,
Chang Gung University, School of Medicine,Taipei, Taiwan

Abstract

Thrombomodulin (TM) is a thrombin-binding anticoagulant cofactor, which is extensively expressed on the surface of endothelial cells. Human TM is a single-chain type 1 transmembrane glycoprotein containing five extracellular domains. TM is an important endogenous anti-coagulant protein. Thrombin-TM complexes transform the inactive from of protein C into an activated protein C (APC). APC subsequently inactivate the coagulation factors Va and VIIIa, thereby suppressing further thrombin generation. In addition, TM also plays an important role in attenuation of inflammatory responses through inhibition of leukocyte adhesion to endothelial cells, inhibition of complement pathways, neutralization of lipopolysaccharide (LPS) as well as sequestration and degradation of pro-inflammatory high-mobility group box 1 protein (HMGB1). Thus, the endothelial surface bounded TM prevents dissemination of pro-coagulant

* Professor Han-Pin Kuo, 199 Tun Hwa N. Rd., Taipei, Taiwan. Email: q8828@ms11.hinet.net.

and pro-inflammatory molecules and allows these molecules to act locally at the site of injury. In patients with sepsis and disseminated intravascular coagulation (DIC), TM expression is down regulated resulting in dissemination of pro-coagulant and pro-inflammatory molecules throughout the systemic circulation. The dual ability of TM to suppress both coagulation and inflammation makes this molecule a possible drug candidate for the treatment for DIC. A soluble form of recombinant human TM (rhsTM) has been shown to be more effective and safer than heparin in treatment of patients with DIC. In fact, rhsTM has been approved for the treatment of DIC in Japan. This chapter focuses on the critical roles of TM in the cross talk between inflammation and coagulation. Furthermore, this chapter provides a rationale for the clinical application of TM for treatment of DIC.

Keywords: Thrombomodulin; disseminated intravascular coagulation; thrombin; activated protein C; coagulant factor; sepsis

Introduction

Disseminated intravascular coagulation (DIC), characterized by systemic activation of intravascular coagulation, has been reported to play an important role in the development of multi-organ failure and death [1]. DIC is associated with the formation of a large number of microthrombotic foci, leading to organ microcirculation failures and subsequent complete organ failure. The formation of diffuse microthrombi in the circulation is followed by thrombolysis in the systemic circulation, leading to the consumption of coagulation factors and platelets [2-4]. The consumption of both platelets and coagulation factors results in thrombocytopenia, a deficiency of coagulation factors, and a bleeding tendency. DIC induced coagulopathy may be modified in the presence of neutrophil proteases and fibrinolysis inhibitors [5, 6]. The development of DIC is exclusively secondary to certain underlying disorders [7]. DIC may be induced by sepsis or major trauma through the activation of a systemic inflammatory response, leading to activation of the cytokine network and subsequent activation of coagulation [2]. In addition, the release or exposure of pro-coagulant material into the bloodstream by malignancy or obstetrical disorders may also be associated with the development of DIC. The outcomes of DIC are mainly related to the underlying diseases and associated complications [7]. However, DIC alone may have a direct impact on mortality of patients. The mortality rate in patients with DIC is higher than those without

DIC, and treatment of DIC reduces the mortality of patients with DIC [7, 8]. Therefore, specific treatment directly against DIC may provide a complementary benefit in improving the prognosis of patients with DIC, when appropriate therapy for the underlying diseases has been implemented.

Thrombomodulin (TM) is a membrane-bound glycoprotein initially identified on vascular endothelium [9], and later on leucocytes, smooth muscle cell, platelet, and cardiomyocyte [10, 11]. TM is also expressed in some cancer cells and influences cancer growth and metastasis [12, 13]. TM protein has 557 amino acids, and its structure consists of 5 domains including a highly charged N-terminal lectin-like domain (D1), a domain with six epidermal growth factor (EGF)-like structures (D2), a serine and threonine-rich domain (D3), a transmembrane domain (D4) and a cytoplasmic domain (D5) [14]. TM was discovered by its anticoagulant activity, to be an essential co-factor for thrombin mediated activation of Protein C [15] and thrombin-activated fibrinolysis inhibitor (TAFI) [16]. Through these mechanisms, the function of TM as a natural anticoagulant has been well documented. TM is also involved in the process of inflammation. TM modifies the inflammatory response [17], prevents leucocyte infiltration [18], suppresses complement system [19], and interferes the effects of high mobility group box 1 (HMGB1) [20].

Once bound to endothelial thrombin, TM accelerates protein C activation and soluble TM (sTM) is released into the serum by proteolytic degradation [21]. sTM is released from the surfaces of endothelial cells after injury only; no other stimulation can trigger it [22]. Therefore, as a marker of endothelial injury, a decrease in endothelial surface expression of TM has been demonstrated in patients with sepsis [23], and sTM levels are elevated in diseases associated with DIC [24]. The elevated serum sTM levels in sepsis-induced DIC regress concomitantly with resolution of DIC [24]. The extent of endothelial injury, as quantified by sTM, independently predicted the development of DIC and mortality in septic patients [24]. In DIC patients, the surface expression of TM may be inadequate after extensive shedding of the membrane-bound TM into soluble serum TM. With regards to the anti-coagulant and anti-inflammatory properties of TM, supply of TM in patents with DIC may provide clinical benefits in these patients. However, the sTM activity is 30% to 50% compared with that of membrane- associated TM. Recently, a soluble form of recombinant human TM (rhsTM), with full activity compared with membrane-bound TM, has been developed in treatment of patients with DIC [25]. This chapter focuses on the critical roles of TM in the cross talk between inflammation and coagulation. This chapter also discusses about the rationale and effectiveness for the clinical application of rhsTM in treatment of DIC.

Anti-coagulant Effects of TM

The anticoagulant effect of TM is mediated through inhibiting thrombin activity. Thrombin is a natural pro-coagulant factor. It activates coagulation factors V, VIII, XI, and XIII. Thrombin has the ability to activate fibrinogen to generate fibrin and also activates platelets. However, the thrombin affinity to pro-coagulant substrates is remarkably reduced by TM binding [26-29]. TM directly inhibits most of the pro-coagulant activities of thrombin including fibrinogen clotting, platelet activation, and factor V activation [26, 27].

The anticoagulant activity of TM is also attributed to enhancing activated protein C (APC) generation. Thrombin-TM complexes transform the inactive form of protein C into activated protein C. APC subsequently inactivates coagulation factors Va and VIIIa, thereby suppressing further thrombin generation. Owing to high expression on the surface of endothelial cells, TM is essential in preventing intravascular thrombus formation. An animal study has revealed that endothelium-specific loss of TM in mice causes spontaneous and fatal thrombosis in the arterial as well as venous circulation [30]; 40% of mutant mice died before birth, and the remaining 60% died within a month after birth because of massive thrombosis. In humans, the endothelial TM expression is down regulated in certain pathologic conditions, such as meningococcal sepsis and graft rejection, resulting in thrombotic complications [23, 31, 32]. Taken together, TM directly binds to thrombin to inhibit its pro-coagulant activity; the TM-thrombin complex further inhibits thrombin generation through activation of APC. A deficiency in TM may cause extensive thrombosis formation (Figure 1).

TM and Inflammation

APC-dependent Mechanism

Increasing lines of evidence have suggested that TM plays an important role in anti-inflammatory effects through APC-dependent and independent mechanisms (Figure 2). APC induced by TM-thrombin complexes prevents inflammation-induced vascular permeability [33, 34], suppresses inflammatory cytokine production in sepsis [35], inhibits leukocyte adhesion, and decreases leukocyte chemotaxis [36]. The anti-inflammatory effects of APC are mediated via endothelial protein C receptor (EPCR) to activate the protease-activated receptor 1 (PAR-1) and its downstream sphingosine-1 phosphate receptor 1 signaling pathway [33].

APC-independent Mechanisms

Thrombin is a potent stimulus of inflammatory reaction. The pro-inflammatory effects of thrombin decreases after binding to TM. Thrombin disrupts the endothelial cell junction and increases tumor necrosis factor alpha production from monocytes [37]. It facilitates the recruitment of circulating monocytes by increasing endothelial expression of monocyte chemoattractant protein-1 (MCP-1), intercellular adhesion molecule-1 (ICAM-1) and vascular cell adhesion molecule-1 (VCAM-1) [38, 39]. The signaling pathway of thrombin is also via PAR-1 activation, but its downstream effector is coupled to the sphingosine-1 phosphate receptor 3.

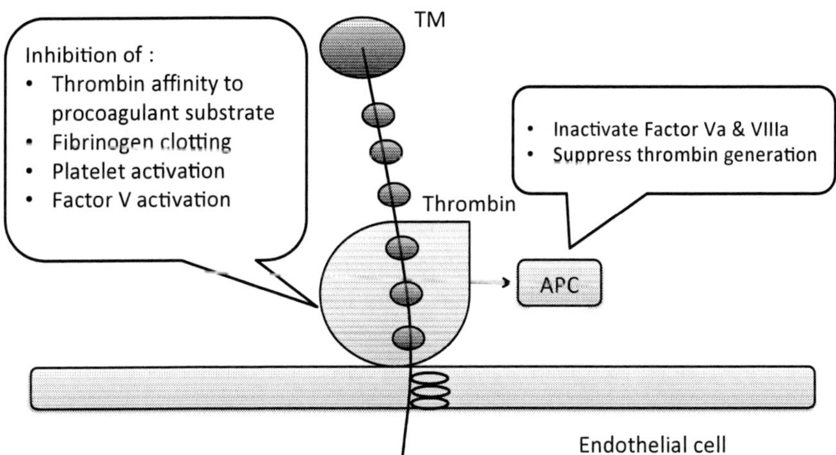

Figure 1. The anticoagulant activities of TM. Thrombin-TM complex activates activated protein C (APC). APC prevents thrombin generation and inactivates factor Va and VIIIa. The thrombin affinity to procoagulant substrates is remarkably reduced by TM binding. TM directly inhibits thrombin included fibrinogen clotting, platelet activation, and factor V activation.

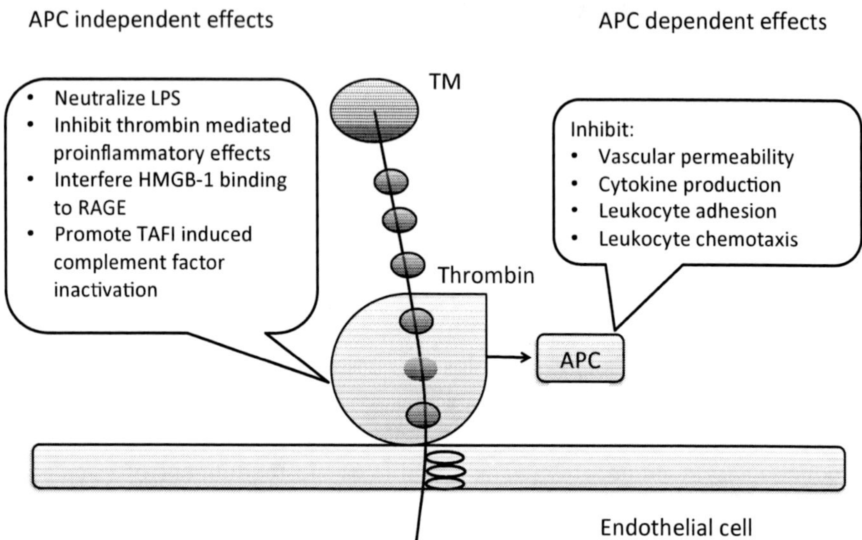

Figure 2. The anti-inflammatory activities of TM. TM attenuates inflammatory responses through APC dependent and independent mechanisms. The activation of APC by thrombin-TM complex causes APC-dependent cytoprotection effects. TM also exerts anti-inflammatory effects through neutralization of lipopolysaccharide (LPS), inhibition of complement system, and interference with high mobility group box 1 (HMGB-1) binding to its receptor; receptor for advanced glycation end products (RAGE).

TM inhibits the interaction of thrombin with PAR-1, and decreases thrombin-induced pro-inflammatory effects. Thereafter, apart from APC/EPCR/PAR1/sphingosine-1 phosphate receptor 1 pathway, TM also plays a pivotal role in regulating thrombin/PAR1/sphingosine-1 phosphate receptor 3 pathways to inhibit inflammation [40].

Thrombin-TM complex activates thrombin activatable fibrinolysis inhibitor (TAFI) [41-43]. TAFI is a circulating zymogen that degrades bradykinin and complement factors C3a and C5a. Complement system is one of the important effectors in human immunity. Excessive activation of the complement system leads to several inflammatory diseases. The thrombin-TM complex activates TAFI with a catalytic efficiency of 1000-fold better than free thrombin alone. TAFI cleaves carboxyl terminal arginines of complement factors and bradykinin, inactivating their biological activities and down-regulating the associated inflammatory reaction [44]. In an animal study, mice lacking the D1 domain of TM display enhanced deposition of complement factor C3 on their joint surfaces and develop more severe inflammatory arthritis than wild-type counterparts [19].

TM may also attenuate inflammation by binding and neutralizing lipopolysaccharide (LPS). TMD1 domain specifically binds to Lewis Y antigen in LPS of gram-negative bacteria [36]. LPS, a component of the cell wall of gram-negative bacteria, provides a potent signal to the innate immune system and is often used to model gram-negative infections *in vitro* and *in vivo*. LPS interacts with CD14 and toll-like receptor on the cell surface and transduces signals from the cell membrane into the cytosol, activating the downstream pro-inflammatory signaling pathways [45]. Soluble TMD1 or recombinant TMD1 (rTMD1) could directly bind to LPS, block the interaction of LPS with CD14 and reduce the subsequent LPS-induced inflammatory reaction by suppressing the activation of mitogen-activated protein kinase and nuclear factor kappa B signaling pathways. The release of pro-inflammatory cytokines and expression of inducible nitric oxide synthase are thereby decreased [46]. By binding to the Lewis Y antigen, rTMD1 can specifically induce the agglutination of *Klebsiella pneumoniae* and enhance the phagocytosis of the bacteria by macrophages [46].

HMGB1 is another anti-inflammatory target of TM. HMGB1 is a ubiquitously expressed nuclear protein that is released from necrotic cells. HMGB1 binds to the receptor for advanced glycation end products (RAGE) and activates the downstream signaling that is implicated in the pathogenesis and/or progression of various clinical disorders, such as infections, sepsis, arthritis, and cancer [47]. The lectin-like domain of TM interferes with HMGB1 binding to RAGE, thereby impairing HMGB1-RAGE signaling [20]. Alternatively, TM may antagonize HMGB1 by enhancing thrombin-mediated proteolytic degradation of HMGB1 [48].

Recombinant TM for Treatment of DIC

The recombinant human soluble TM (rhsTM) derived from Chinese hamster ovary (CHO) cells, is composed of the extracellular domain of TM [49]. Similar to membrane-bound native TM, rhsTM retains the ability to bind to thrombin and APC. Administration of rhsTM has been shown to protect rats from tissue factor and endotoxin-induced DIC or lung injury [50-52]. In addition, rhsTM not only reduces compression trauma-induced spinal cord injury by inhibiting leukocyte accumulation and expression of TNF-α [53], but also provides protection against ischemia-reperfusion injury in the liver and kidney [54, 55].

The rhsTM was first introduced in Japan after the success of a multicenter, randomized, double-blinded, phase 3 study involving 232 patients with DIC complicated hematological malignancies (n = 131) or infection (n = 101) [25]. This clinical trial was designed to compare rhsTM (0.06 mg/kg for 30min once day) with heparin (8U/kg/h for 24 h) in DIC patients. The primary end point was DIC resolution rate at day 7, and the secondary end points were disappearance rate of bleeding symptoms at day 7 and 28-day mortality rates. The DIC resolution rate at day 7 was significantly better in patients receiving rhsTM (66.1%) than in those receiving heparin (49.9%). The disappearance rate of bleeding symptoms at day 7 was also better in patients receiving rhsTM (35.2%) than in those receiving heparin (20.9%). However, the 28-day mortality of patients receiving rhsTM treatment did not differ from patients receiving heparin treatment both in DIC resulting from infection (rhsTM 28.0%; heparin 34.6%), and DIC resulting from hematologic malignancy (rhsTM 17.2%; heparin 18.0%). Greater decreases in plasma thrombin-antithrombin complex levels and D-dimer levels were observed in patients treated with rhsTM. Importantly, rhsTM treatment showed a better safety profile with a lower incidence of bleeding-related adverse events.

A retrospective subanalysis on 80 patients with infection associated DIC reveals a similar DIC resolution rate (rhsTM: 67.5%; heparin: 55.6%) and 28-day mortality rate (rhsTM: 21.4%; heparin: 31.6%) [56]. However, the 28-day mortality rate is significantly lower for patients in whom DIC resolved (8.5%, P= 0.0004) than those in whom DIC did not resolve (44.8%). Patients in whom DIC resolved with rhsTM treatment had lower 28-day mortality rate (3.7%), compared to those in whom DIC with heparin treatment (15%).

A recent study using propensity score retrospectively analyzed 162 patients with sepsis-induced DIC [57]. Among them, 68 patients received rhsTM and the other 94 patients received heparin (15%), antithrombin (7%) or no specific treatment for DIC (78%). After adjusting for these imbalances by stratified propensity score analysis, rhTM treatment was significantly associated with reduced in-hospital mortality (40% vs. 57%; adjusted hazard ratio, 0.45; 95 % confidential interval, 0.26–0.77; p = 0.013). An association between rhTM treatment and higher numbers of intensive care unit-free days, ventilator-free days, and vasopressor-free days were also observed. DIC scores were significantly decreased in the rhTM group compared with the control group in the early period of treatment, whereas the incidence of bleeding related adverse events was not different between two groups.

A post-marketing surveillance study was conducted to assess the safety and effectiveness of rhsTM in the treatment of DIC [58], including 2516 DIC patients associated with infection and 1032 patients with hematological malignancy. The DIC scores were significantly decreased in both groups with rhsTM treatment. The incidences of critical bleeding in the infection-associated DIC and malignancy-associated DIC groups were 2.6% and 2.4%, and the survival rates were 64.1% and 70.7%, respectively. This study demonstrates that rhsTM treatment in DIC patients provides effectiveness in DIC resolution and a low incidence of bleeding adverse effect.

In the United States, a phase IIB clinical trial involving 741 patients has been completed by May 2011 to compare the clinical effectiveness of rhsTM in the treatment of sepsis with DIC (NCT00487656). The results of this study have been uploaded on the website (http://www.artisanpharma.net/news.htm.). A Phase III study is currently being conducted in the US for patients with severe sepsis associated DIC (NCT01598831).

Conclusion

The crosstalk between coagulation and inflammation constitutes the critical components of the pathophysiological mechanisms for DIC. TM, expressed on the surface of endothelial cells, prevents activation of pro-coagulant and pro-inflammatory molecules, including thrombin, complement factors, LPS, and HMGB1. However, TM expression is down-regulated in patients with sepsis and DIC, which may result in systemic dissemination of pro-coagulant and pro-inflammatory responses. The ability of TM to suppress both coagulation and inflammation makes this molecule a potential candidate for treatment of DIC. The therapeutic application of rhsTM in patients with DIC has been investigated extensively and rhsTM has been approved in Japan for the treatment of DIC since 2008. To date, rhsTM has been shown effective in resolution of DIC with a relatively reasonable incidence of bleeding adverse effect. However, the effect of rhsTM treatment on mortality of patients with DIC warrants a large scale, randomized, controlled study.

References

[1]   Esmon, C. T., Fukudome, K., Mather, T., Bode, W., Regan, L. M., Stearns-Kurosawa, D. J., Kurosawa, S. (1999). Inflammation, sepsis, and coagulation. *Haematologica*. 84, 254-9.

[2]   Levi, M., Ten Cate, H. (1999). Disseminated intravascular coagulation. *The New England journal of medicine*. 341, 586-92.

[3]   Taylor, F. B., Jr., Toh, C. H., Hoots, W. K., Wada, H., Levi, M. (2001). Towards definition, clinical and laboratory criteria, and a scoring system for disseminated intravascular coagulation. *Thrombosis and haemostasis*. 86, 1327-30.

[4]   Levi, M., Toh, C. H., Thachil, J., Watson, H. G. (2009). Guidelines for the diagnosis and management of disseminated intravascular coagulation. British Committee for Standards in Haematology. *British journal of haematology*. 145, 24-33.

[5]   Ono, T., Mimuro, J., Madoiwa, S., Soejima, K., Kashiwakura, Y., Ishiwata, A., Takano, K., Ohmori, T., Sakata, Y. (2006). Severe secondary deficiency of von Willebrand factor-cleaving protease (ADAMTS13) in patients with sepsis-induced disseminated intravascular coagulation: its correlation with development of renal failure. *Blood*. 107, 528-34.

[6]   Madoiwa, S., Tanaka, H., Nagahama, Y., Dokai, M., Kashiwakura, Y., Ishiwata, A., Sakata, A., Yasumoto, A., Ohmori, T., Mimuro, J., Sakata, Y. (2011). Degradation of cross-linked fibrin by leukocyte elastase as alternative pathway for plasmin-mediated fibrinolysis in sepsis-induced disseminated intravascular coagulation. *Thrombosis research*. 127, 349-55.

[7]   Wada, H., Asakura, H., Okamoto, K., Iba, T., Uchiyama, T., Kawasugi, K., Koga, S., Mayumi, T., Koike, K., Gando, S., Kushimoto, S., Seki, Y., Madoiwa, S., Maruyama, I., Yoshioka, A. (2010). Expert consensus for the treatment of disseminated intravascular coagulation in Japan. *Thrombosis research*. 125, 6-11.

[8]   Kienast, J., Juers, M., Wiedermann, C. J., Hoffmann, J. N., Ostermann, H., Strauss, R., Keinecke, H. O., Warren, B. L., Opal, S. M. (2006). Treatment effects of high-dose antithrombin without concomitant heparin in patients with severe sepsis with or without disseminated intravascular coagulation. *Journal of thrombosis and haemostasis : 4, 90-7.

[9]   Maruyama, I., Bell, C. E., Majerus, P. W. (1985). Thrombomodulin is found on endothelium of arteries, veins, capillaries, and lymphatics, and on syncytiotrophoblast of human placenta. *The Journal of cell biology*. 101, 363-71.

[10] McCachren, S. S., Diggs, J., Weinberg, J. B., Dittman, W. A. (1991). Thrombomodulin expression by human blood monocytes and by human synovial tissue lining macrophages. *Blood.* 78, 3128-32.

[11] Tohda, G., Oida, K., Okada, Y., Kosaka, S., Okada, E., Takahashi, S., Ishii, H., Miyamori, I. (1998). Expression of thrombomodulin in atherosclerotic lesions and mitogenic activity of recombinant thrombomodulin in vascular smooth muscle cells. *Arteriosclerosis, thrombosis, and vascular biology.* 18, 1861-9.

[12] Zhang, Y., Weiler-Guettler, H., Chen, J., Wilhelm, O., Deng, Y., Qiu, F., Nakagawa, K., Klevesath, M., Wilhelm, S., Bohrer, H., Nakagawa, M., Graeff, H., Martin, E., Stern, D. M., Rosenberg, R. D., Ziegler, R., Nawroth, P. P. (1998). Thrombomodulin modulates growth of tumor cells independent of its anticoagulant activity. *The Journal of clinical investigation.* 101, 1301-9.

[13] Horowitz, N. A., Blevins, E. A., Miller, W. M., Perry, A. R., Talmage, K. E., Mullins, E. S., Flick, M. J., Queiroz, K. C., Shi, K., Spek, C. A., Conway, E. M., Monia, B. P., Weiler, H., Degen, J. L., Palumbo, J. S. (2011). Thrombomodulin is a determinant of metastasis through a mechanism linked to the thrombin binding domain but not the lectin-like domain. *Blood.* 118, 2889-95.

[14] Suzuki, K., Kusumoto, H., Deyashiki, Y., Nishioka, J., Maruyama, I., Zushi, M., Kawahara, S., Honda, G., Yamamoto, S., Horiguchi, S. (1987). Structure and expression of human thrombomodulin, a thrombin receptor on endothelium acting as a cofactor for protein C activation. *The EMBO journal.* 6, 1891-7.

[15] Esmon, C. T. (1989). The roles of protein C and thrombomodulin in the regulation of blood coagulation. *The Journal of biological chemistry.* 264, 4743-6.

[16] de Munk, G. A., Groeneveld, E., Rijken, D. C. (1991). Acceleration of the thrombin inactivation of single chain urokinase-type plasminogen activator (pro-urokinase) by thrombomodulin. *The Journal of clinical investigation.* 88, 1680-4. 10.1172/JCI115483.

[17] Weiler, H., Lindner, V., Kerlin, B., Isermann, B. H., Hendrickson, S. B., Cooley, B. C., Meh, D. A., Mosesson, M. W., Shworak, N. W., Post, M. J., Conway, E. M., Ulfman, L. H., von Andrian, U. H., Weitz, J. I. (2001). Characterization of a mouse model for thrombomodulin deficiency. *Arteriosclerosis, thrombosis, and vascular biology.* 21, 1531-7.

[18] Ikeguchi, H., Maruyama, S., Morita, Y., Fujita, Y., Kato, T., Natori, Y., Akatsu, H., Campbell, W., Okada, N., Okada, H., Yuzawa, Y., Matsuo, S. (2002). Effects of human soluble thrombomodulin on experimental glomerulonephritis. *Kidney international.* 61, 490-501.

[19] Van de Wouwer, M., Plaisance, S., De Vriese, A., Waelkens, E., Collen, D., Persson, J., Daha, M. R., Conway, E. M. (2006). The lectin-like domain of thrombomodulin interferes with complement activation and protects against arthritis. *Journal of thrombosis and haemostasis :* 4, 1813-24.

[20] Abeyama, K., Stern, D. M., Ito, Y., Kawahara, K., Yoshimoto, Y., Tanaka, M., Uchimura. T., Ida, N., Yamazaki, Y., Yamada, S., Yamamoto, Y., Yamamoto, H., Iino, S., Taniguchi, N., Maruyama, I. (2005). The N-terminal domain of thrombomodulin sequesters high-mobility group-B1 protein, a novel antiinflammatory mechanism. *The Journal of clinical investigation.* 115, 1267-74.

[21] Takano, S., Kimura, S., Ohdama, S., Aoki, N. (1990). Plasma thrombomodulin in health and diseases. *Blood.* 76, 2024-9.

[22] Boehme, M. W., Galle, P., Stremmel, W. (2002). Kinetics of thrombomodulin release and endothelial cell injury by neutrophil-derived proteases and oxygen radicals. *Immunology.* 107, 340-9.

[23] Faust, S. N., Levin, M., Harrison, O. B., Goldin, R. D., Lockhart, M. S., Kondaveeti, S., Laszik, Z., Esmon, C. T., Heyderman, R. S. (2001). Dysfunction of endothelial protein C activation in severe meningococcal sepsis. *The New England journal of medicine.* 345, 408-16.

[24] Lin, S. M., Wang, Y. M., Lin, H. C., Lee, K. Y., Huang, C. D., Liu, C. Y., Wang, C. H., Kuo, H. P. (2008). Serum thrombomodulin level relates to the clinical course of disseminated intravascular coagulation, multiorgan dysfunction syndrome, and mortality in patients with sepsis. *Critical care medicine.* 36, 683-9.

[25] Saito, H., Maruyama, I., Shimazaki, S., Yamamoto, Y., Aikawa, N., Ohno, R., Hirayama, A., Matsuda, T., Asakura, H., Nakashima, M., Aoki, N. (2007). Efficacy and safety of recombinant human soluble thrombomodulin (ART-123) in disseminated intravascular coagulation: results of a phase III, randomized, double-blind clinical trial. *Journal of thrombosis and haemostasis :* 5, 31-41.

[26] Esmon, N. L., Carroll, R. C., Esmon, C. T. (1983). Thrombomodulin blocks the ability of thrombin to activate platelets. *The Journal of biological chemistry.* 258, 12238-42.

[27] Esmon, C. T., Esmon, N. L., Harris, K. W. (1982). Complex formation between thrombin and thrombomodulin inhibits both thrombin-catalyzed fibrin formation and factor V activation. *The Journal of biological chemistry*. 257, 7944-7.

[28] Esmon, C. T. (1993). Molecular events that control the protein C anticoagulant pathway. *Thrombosis and haemostasis*. 70, 29-35.

[29] Castellino, F. J. (1995). Human protein C and activated protein C Components of the human anticoagulation system. *Trends in cardiovascular medicine*. 5, 55-62.

[30] Isermann, B., Hendrickson, S. B., Zogg, M., Wing, M., Cummiskey, M., Kisanuki, Y. Y., Yanagisawa, M., Weiler, H. (2001). Endothelium-specific loss of murine thrombomodulin disrupts the protein C anticoagulant pathway and causes juvenile-onset thrombosis. *The Journal of clinical investigation*. 108, 537-46.

[31] Tsuchida, A., Salem, H., Thomson, N., Hancock, W. W. (1992). Tumor necrosis factor production during human renal allograft rejection is associated with depression of plasma protein C and free protein S levels and decreased intragraft thrombomodulin expression. *The Journal of experimental medicine*. 175, 81-90.

[32] Iino, S., Abeyama, K., Kawahara, K. I,, Aikou, T., Maruyama, I. (2004). Thrombomodulin expression on Langerhans' islet: can endogenous 'anticoagulant on demand' overcome detrimental thrombotic complications in clinical islet transplantation? *Journal of thrombosis and haemostasis* : 2, 833-4.

[33] Feistritzer, C., Riewald, M. (2005). Endothelial barrier protection by activated protein C through PAR1-dependent sphingosine 1-phosphate receptor-1 crossactivation. *Blood*. 105, 3178-84.

[34] Schucpbach, R. A., Feistritzer, C., Fernandez, J. A., Griffin, J. H., Riewald, M. (2009). Protection of vascular barrier integrity by activated protein C in murine models depends on protease-activated receptor-1. *Thrombosis and haemostasis*. 101, 724-33.

[35] Murakami, K., Okajima, K., Uchiba, M., Johno, M., Nakagaki, T., Okabe, H., Takatsuki, K. (1997). Activated protein C prevents LPS-induced pulmonary vascular injury by inhibiting cytokine production. *The American journal of physiology*. 272, L197-202.

[36] Hirose, K., Okajima, K., Taoka, Y., Uchiba, M., Tagami, H., Nakano, K., Utoh, J., Okabe, H., Kitamura, N. (2000). Activated protein C reduces the ischemia/reperfusion-induced spinal cord injury in rats by inhibiting neutrophil activation. *Annals of surgery*. 232, 272-80.

[37] Rabiet, M. J., Plantier, J. L., Rival, Y., Genoux, Y., Lampugnani, M. G., Dejana, E. (1996). Thrombin-induced increase in endothelial permeability is associated with changes in cell-to-cell junction organization. *Arteriosclerosis, thrombosis, and vascular biology.* 16, 488-96.

[38] Colotta, F., Sciacca, F. L., Sironi, M., Luini, W., Rabiet, M. J., Mantovani, A. (1994). Expression of monocyte chemotactic protein-1 by monocytes and endothelial cells exposed to thrombin. *The American journal of pathology.* 144, 975-85.

[39] Kaplanski, G., Marin, V., Fabrigoule, M., Boulay, V., Benoliel, A. M., Bongrand, P., Kaplanski, S., Farnarier, C. (1998). Thrombin-activated human endothelial cells support monocyte adhesion in vitro following expression of intercellular adhesion molecule-1 (ICAM-1; CD54) and vascular cell adhesion molecule-1 (VCAM-1; CD106). *Blood.* 92, 1259-67.

[40] Ruf, W., Furlan-Freguia, C., Niessen, F. (2009). Vascular and dendritic cell coagulation signaling in sepsis progression. *Journal of thrombosis and haemostasis.* 7 Suppl 1, 118-21.

[41] Campbell, W., Okada, N., Okada, H. (2001). Carboxypeptidase R is an inactivator of complement-derived inflammatory peptides and an inhibitor of fibrinolysis. *Immunological reviews.* 180, 162-7.

[42] Nishimura, T., Myles, T., Piliponsky, A. M., Kao, P. N., Berry, G. J., Leung, L. L. (2007). Thrombin-activatable procarboxypeptidase B regulates activated complement C5a in vivo. *Blood.* 109, 1992-7.

[43] Delvaeye, M., Noris, M., De Vriese, A., Esmon, C. T., Esmon, N. L., Ferrell, G., Del-Favero, J., Plaisance, S., Claes, B., Lambrechts, D., Zoja, C., Remuzzi, G., Conway, E. M. (2009). Thrombomodulin mutations in atypical hemolytic-uremic syndrome. *The New England journal of medicine.* 361, 345-57.

[44] Leung, L. L., Myles, T., Nishimura, T., Song, J. J., Robinson, W. H. (2008). Regulation of tissue inflammation by thrombin-activatable carboxypeptidase B (or TAFI). *Molecular immunology.* 45, 4080-3.

[45] Lin, S. M., Frevert, C. W., Kajikawa, O., Wurfel, M. M., Ballman, K., Mongovin, S., Wong, V. A., Selk, A., Martin, T. R. (2004). Differential regulation of membrane CD14 expression and endotoxin-tolerance in alveolar macrophages. *American journal of respiratory cell and molecular biology.* 31, 162-70.

[46] Shi, C. S., Shi, G. Y., Hsiao, S. M., Kao, Y. C., Kuo, K. L., Ma, C. Y., Kuo, C. H., Chang, B. I., Chang, C. F., Lin, C. H., Wong, C. H., Wu, H.

L. (2008). Lectin-like domain of thrombomodulin binds to its specific ligand Lewis Y antigen and neutralizes lipopolysaccharide-induced inflammatory response. *Blood.* 112, 3661-70.

[47] Lotze, M. T., Tracey, K. J. (2005). High-mobility group box 1 protein (HMGB1): nuclear weapon in the immune arsenal. *Nature reviews Immunology.* 5, 331-42.

[48] Ito, T., Kawahara, K., Okamoto, K., Yamada, S., Yasuda, M., Imaizumi, H., Nawa, Y., Meng, X., Shrestha, B., Hashiguchi, T., Maruyama, I. (2008). Proteolytic cleavage of high mobility group box 1 protein by thrombin-thrombomodulin complexes. *Arteriosclerosis, thrombosis, and vascular biology.* 28, 1825-30.

[49] Gomi, K., Zushi, M., Honda, G., Kawahara, S., Matsuzaki, O., Kanabayashi, T., Yamamoto, S., Maruyama, I., Suzuki, K. (1990). Antithrombotic effect of recombinant human thrombomodulin on thrombin-induced thromboembolism in mice. *Blood.* 75, 1396-9.

[50] Gonda, Y., Hirata, S., Saitoh, K., Aoki, Y., Mohri, M., Gomi, K., Sugihara, T., Kiyota, T., Yamamoto, S., Ishida, T., et al. (1993). Antithrombotic effect of recombinant human soluble thrombomodulin on endotoxin-induced disseminated intravascular coagulation in rats. *Thrombosis research.* 71, 325-35.

[51] Mohri, M., Oka, M., Aoki, Y., Gonda, Y., Hirata, S., Gomi, K., Kiyota, T., Sugihara, T., Yamamoto, S., Ishida, T., et al. (1994). Intravenous extended infusion of recombinant human soluble thrombomodulin prevented tissue factor-induced disseminated intravascular coagulation in rats. *American journal of hematology.* 45, 298-303.

[52] Uchiba, M., Okajima, K., Murakami, K., Nawa, K., Okabe, H., Takatsuki, K. (1995). ecombinant human soluble thrombomodulin reduces endotoxin-induced pulmonary vascular injury via protein C activation in rats. *Thrombosis and haemostasis.* 74, 1265-70.

[53] Taoka, Y., Okajima, K., Uchiba, M., Johno, M. (2000). Neuroprotection by recombinant thrombomodulin. *Thrombosis and haemostasis.* 83, 462-8.

[54] Kaneko, H., Joubara, N., Yoshino, M., Yamazaki, K., Mitumaru, A., Miki, Y., Satake, H., Shiba, T. (2000). Protective effect of human urinary thrombomodulin on ischemia- reperfusion injury in the canine liver. *European surgical research Europaische chirurgische Forschung Recherches chirurgicales europeennes.* 32, 87-93. 8745.

[55] Ozaki, T., Anas, C., Maruyama, S., Yamamoto, T., Yasuda, K., Morita, Y., Ito, Y., Gotoh, M., Yuzawa, Y., Matsuo, S. (2008). Intrarenal

administration of recombinant human soluble thrombomodulin ameliorates ischaemic acute renal failure. *Nephrology, dialysis, transplantation : official publication of the European Dialysis and Transplant Association - European Renal Association.* 23, 110-9.

[56] Aikawa, N., Shimazaki, S., Yamamoto, Y., Saito, H., Maruyama, I., Ohno, R., Hirayama, A., Aoki, Y., Aoki, N. (2011). Thrombomodulin alfa in the treatment of infectious patients complicated by disseminated intravascular coagulation: subanalysis from the phase 3 trial. *Shock.* 35, 349-54.

[57] Yamakawa, K., Ogura, H., Fujimi, S., Morikawa, M., Ogawa, Y., Mohri, T., Nakamori, Y., Inoue, Y., Kuwagata, Y., Tanaka, H., Hamasaki, T., Shimazu, T. (2013). Recombinant human soluble thrombomodulin in sepsis-induced disseminated intravascular coagulation: a multicenter propensity score analysis. *Intensive care medicine.* 39, 644-52.

[58] Mimuro, J., Takahashi, H., Kitajima, I., Tsuji, H., Eguchi, Y., Matsushita, T., Kuroda, T., Sakata, Y. (2013). Impact of recombinant soluble thrombomodulin (thrombomodulin alfa) on disseminated intravascular coagulation. *Thrombosis research.* 10.1016/ j.thromres.2013.03.008.

In: Disseminated Intravascular Coagulation (DIC)   ISBN: 978-1-62948-323-8
Editor: Balwinder Singh   © 2014 Nova Science Publishers, Inc.

Chapter IV

Diagnostic Scoring System for Disseminated Intravascular Coagulation

R. K. Singh, MD[*]
Department of Critical Care Medicine, Sanjay Gandhi Post Graduate
Institute of Medical Sciences (SGPGIMS), Lucknow, Uttar Pradesh, India

Abstract

Disseminated intravascular coagulation (DIC) is an acquired
syndrome characterized by intravascular activation of coagulation as a
result of varied etiology. DIC in itself is associated with increased
morbidity and mortality. Rapid diagnosis of DIC is highly desirable as
prompt initiation of treatment may improve outcomes. However, since no
single clinical or laboratory test has an adequate sensitivity and
specificity to confirm or reject diagnosis of DIC, there's need to
incorporate both clinical and laboratory parameters into one composite
scoring system for the diagnosis of DIC. Scoring systems to diagnose
DIC were developed by Japanese Ministry of Health and Welfare

[*] Corresponding author: Dr. Ratender K. Singhi, Sanjay Gandhi Post Graduate Institute of
Medical Sciences (SGPGIMS), Lucknow, Uttar Pradesh, India. E-mail: ratender@sgpgi.ac.
in.

(JMHW) in 1988, International Society of Thrombosis and Hemostasis (ISTH) in 2001 and by Japanese Association for Acute Medicine (JAAM) in 2006.

Each of these scores have unique attributes applicable to some but not all etiologies of DIC. The utility of a specific DIC score is dictated by the purpose (treatment or diagnosis) for which it is to be used. In a dynamic condition like DIC serial monitoring via these scores may be more useful for both diagnosis and prognosis. In the near future hemostatic molecular markers with higher sensitivity and specificity may circumvent the limitations of the existing DIC scores.

Keywords: Disseminated intravascular coagulation. Diagnostic score

Introduction

Disseminated intravascular coagulation (DIC) is an ominous complication arising from varied conditions like infection, trauma, and malignancy [1-3].

In 2001, international society of thrombosis and homeostasis, scientific subcommittee (ISTH/SSC) defined DIC as "an acquired syndrome characterized by intravascular activation of coagulation with loss of localization arising from different causes. It can originate from or cause damage to the microvasculature, which if sufficiently severe can produce organ dysfunction" [4].

In sepsis, the vicious cycle of vascular endothelial cell damage and associated intravascular fibrin formation arises from cross talk between coagulation and inflammation [5]. Though bleeding and organ dysfunction are both manifestations of DIC, it is the former which attracts more attention despite being a late manifeststion. In DIC of septic origin, organ dysfunction occurs due to microvascular thrombi, angiogenic factors, hyperendotoxemia, and hypercytokinemia [6, 7, 8].

Rapid diagnosis and prompt initiation of treatment with interventions directed against both coagulation and inflammation have been shown to improve outcomes in DIC associated with severe sepsis [9, 10].

Diagnosis of DIC

Currently, gold standard diagnostic test for DIC does not exist. No single clinical or laboratory test has an adequate sensitivity and specificity to confirm or reject the diagnosis of DIC. Screening assays (global coagulation tests), such as the prothrombin time (PT), fibrinogen, platelet count, and fibrin-related markers (FRMs), provide important evidence of the degree of coagulation factor activation and consumption. However, it is important to remember that the underlying diseases which cause DIC, also interfere with the interpretation of several tests used for its diagnosis. Though sensitive, a prolonged PT and or a declining platelet count in serial estimations, are non-specific signs of DIC [11, 12]. Contrary to this fibrinogen is specific, but with poor sensitivity. Low levels of fibrinogen are indicative of the late severe consumptive stage of DIC, prior to which it remain falsely normal or even high [13]. Thus despite it's diagnostic significance [12], hypofibrinogenemia is uncommon except in the most severe cases of DIC. Elevated FRMs, such as fibrinogen and fibrin degradation products (FDPs) [14], D-dimer [15], and soluble fibrin (SF) are all ndices of thrombin formation. However, these and biphasic APTT waveform standalone have not found wide spread clinical acceptability for diagnosis of DIC. Furthermore, elevated FRMs may also be occur in trauma, recent surgery, or venous thromboembolism. Hence, existing guidelines recommend combination of various laboratory markers as against a single marker for diagnosis of DIC [12, 16, 17].

Numerous hemostatic molecular markers with higher sensitivity (but with lower specificity) may be useful in diagnosis of DIC. However, at present constraints of cost, clinical bed side ready availiability and, poorly defined cut offs hamper their wide spread clinical use.

Scoring Systems

As impractical as it may seem, we ideally need a unique DIC score for each of the underlying diseases that cause DIC. Absence of an unquestionable diagnostic standard for DIC, will continue to fuel research and validation in search for an ideal diagnostic score with equally high sensitivity and specifcity, clinical bed-side easy applicability, ready availablity, and suitability for a wide array of DIC causing diseases. Scoring systems to diagnose DIC were developed by Japanese Ministry of Health and Welfare (JMHW) in 1988 [18] from its older 1983 criteria [19], ISTH/SSC in 2001 [4], and by Japanese Association for Acute Medicine (JAAM) in 2006 [20]. All three consist of assays of global markers of coagulation and fibrinolysis that are commonly available in all hospitals.

ISTH/SSC further categorized DIC into an overt (decompenasted), and non-overt (pre-DIC or compensated) DIC. The British Committee for Standards in Hematology (BCSH), the Japanese Society of Thrombosis and Hemostasis (JSTH), and the Italian Society for Thrombosis and Hemostasis (SISET) have all recommended their use for diagnosis of DIC [16, 17, 21]. The JMHW and ISTH overt DIC diagnostic scoring system, are considered the first-generation DIC score, the JAAM DIC score (involving global coagulation tests and their changes) is considered the second-generation score, while those including non-overt DIC diagnostic score (involving global coagulation tests, changes in these tests and hemostatic molecular markers) as the third-generation DIC diagnostic scoring system [22].

The JMHW DIC Scoring System

The JMHW DIC diagnostic score is as depicted in the table 1. Used exclusively in hematological malignancies (HPT) it has shown moderate sensitivity and high specificity (HPT). It's reliance on subjective clinical symptoms of bleeding and thrombosis induced organ dysfunction for which a a point each is given, compromises its sensitivity compared to the newer DIC diagnostic scoring systems. Differentiation is also made between patients with (HPT+) and without (HPT-) hematopoietic malignancies, such that bleeding symptoms in HPT are given one point and changes in platelet count are not given a score in HPT+ patients. A score of four or more in HPT+ and seven or more in HPT- patients is considered diagnostic for DIC. Table 2 depicts some of its advantages and limitations.

The ISTH DIC Scoring System

The ISTH/SSC overt and non-overt DIC diagnostic scoring system is depicted in the table 1. Prior risk assessment for identification of an underlying clinical condition that may be associated with DIC is mandatory before using the overt DIC score. Also, multiple FRMs (FDP, D-dimer & SF) are used as against FDP alone in JMWH and JAAM DIC scores. A score in excess of five is compatible with diagnosis of overt DIC. A score less than five is suggestive (not affirmative) for non-overt DIC and needs to be repeated in the next one to two days. Briefly summarized in table 2 are some of it's advantages and limitations.

ISTH Overt-DIC Diagnostic Scoring System

The diagnostic criteria of ISTH overt DIC [4] are a modified version of the JMHW DIC score [18]. No points are given for clinical symptoms of bleeding and organ dysfunction due to thrombosis since the DIC score in itself may form part of scores for organ failure. Though objective abnormal laboratory values are used for it's diagnosis, no objective clear cut off values have been defined for FDP and SF. However, for D-dimer a level >4.0 µg/mL is considered a moderate increase, and >40 µg/ mL is a strong increase [24]. These cut off values have also been recommended by the Italian Society for Hemostasis and Thrombosis (SISET) [17]. The ISTH overt DIC score has a higher specificity but lower sensitivity compared to JMHW DIC [18]. In sepsis, severe sepsis, surgery or trauma it possessess acceptable diagnostic accuracy and a higher score relates to a higher mortality [23, 24].

ISTH Non-Overt DIC Diagnostic Scoring System

Poor sensitivity and specificity of global coagulation tests, prevents diagnosis of non-overt DIC. Hemostatic markers like antithrobin (AT), protein-C, and thrombin antithrombin (TAT) complex could diagnose this pre-DIC stage.

In presence of an underlying disease known to be associated with DIC major and specific criteria are to be considered in this scoring system. Similar global coagulation tests are used as in overt-DIC, but with emphasis on trends over time, inorder to increase the sensitivity. The SSC recommends daily measurements. Specific criteria require AT or protein C or TAT complexes etc depending on local availability. However, these criteria were not well established [26-29], and now a few more have also been reported [30]. A prospective study sugested that molecular hemoststic biomarkers like TAT, the fibrin monomer complex (FMC), and AT are useful for diagnosis of pre-DIC [16].

Several definitions of pre-DIC have been proposed including diagnosis within a week before onset of DIC [31], four points of overt DIC scores [4], or a markedly high hemostatic molecular marker profile, among others. Combination of the two ISTH scoring systems [23, 32], or addition of organ failure score to it [33] may improve the diagnostic capabilities of the non-overt DIC scoring system [34].

The JAAM DIC Diagnostic Scoring System

In critically ill, the close association between coagulation and inflammation [36] is evident by the role of systemic inflammatory response syndrome (SIRS) in development of DIC. Realizing that rapid diagnosis and prompt treatment would improve outcomes in DIC, JAAM propsoed a new JAAM DIC score for the critically ill patients [9, 10, 20]. Insufficient diagnostic sensitivity and subjective clinical criteria of the JMWH score stimulated the conception of a new DIC scoring system [20, 35]. In a prospective validation study conducted in thirteen critical care centers of Japan, Gando S, et al., concluded that the JAAM DIC score had an acceptable property for the diagnosis of DIC and could identify most of the patients diagnosed by JMHW and ISTH score [20].

He further proposed that the revised JAAM DIC score (without fibrinogen) would be useful for selecting DIC patients for early treatment in the critical care setting [20]. Both older and revised JAAM DIC scores are depicted in the table 1. A brief summary of advantages and limitations of this score are depicted in table 2. Increased sensitivity of this score for diagnosis of DIC has been shown in critically ill patients [20, 35], trauma [37, 38], and obstetric disorders [39, 40]. It must be emphasized that in sepsis, JAAM DIC exists in a dependent continium with ISTH overt DIC, thus providing guidance for early treatment [35, 41].

Comparisons between the Three DIC Diagnostic Scoring Systems

Absence of a gold standard diagnostic test makes diagnosis of DIC challenging. Combination of readily available tests and clinical parameters into scores have reduced the impediments and thus facilitated the process of DIC diagnosis [16, 17, 21]. However, it must be borne in mind that some degree of arbitrariness in assigning power to individual parameters will be an inherent property of various scoring systems. Moreover, since a single definitive standard diagnostic test for DIC seems a distant possibility, finding the most accurate scoring system is likely to remain a matter of further research and validation. A score with the highest sensitivity and specificity, applicable in majority of DIC causing diseases, and that which can be clincally applied in critically sick population would be universally acceptable. However, at present it wouldn't be inappropriate to say that "one size does not fit all" in the DIC diagnostic scoring systems. A brief summary of the advantages and disadvantages of each of the scores is depicted in Table 2.

ISTH DIC score is often also used in children. In a retrospective analysis in children with sepsis and septic shock, ISTH DIC score early in ICU admission, is associated with higher mortality [50]. However, difference in odds ratio for prediction of outcome in DIC was not observed prospectively with either of the scores, despite the fact that they were related to poor outcomes [51].

It must be reemphasized that, a combination of tests repeated over time in a patient with suspected DIC can be used to diagnose the disorder with reasonable certainity [3, 52, 53]. While the ISTH score has a higher specificity, the JAAM DIC has a higher sensitivity for diagnosis of DIC. JAAM score is more helpful for selecting DIC patients for early treatment. It is important to have a score with higher sensitivity to start early treatment of DIC, but it is also equally important to ensure that no person without DIC receives the treatment. For this a test with highest sensitivity and highest specificity applicable to most DIC causing diseases would be best suited. Comparisons between DIC and non-DIC patients seems a predictable conclusion. However, discriminatin between survivors and non-survivors amongst DIC patients is the challenge. Serial trends and delta changes within DIC scores may provide relevant prognostication [58]. Large prospective muticenter studies aimed at comparing survivors and non-survivors amongst the DIC patients is likely to address this issue.

Conclusion

DIC leads to consumption of platelets and coagulation factors, potentially causing severe bleeding. Exhausted fibrinolytic activity contributes to microcirculatiory fibrin deposits resulting in multiple organ failure. A large number of varied clincal conditions predispose to DIC. It's high mortality and morbidity warrant early diagnosis and prompt treatment. In absence of a diagnostic gold standard, reliance on the three DIC scores continues for both diagnosis and prognosis. However, the search for not only the most sensitive

Table 1. Comparative Summary of DIC Diagnostic Scoring Systems

Scoring System	Japanese Ministry of Health and Welfare (JMHW) DIC score (1988)	International Society of Thrombosis and Hemostasis (ISTH) DIC score (2001)		Japanese Association for Acute Medicine (JAAM) DIC score (2006)	
		Overt DIC score	Non-overt DIC score	JAAM DIC score	Revised JAAM DIC score
Parameter	Parameter Value or Range = Score				
Underlying disease	1	Mandatory Risk assessment If yes: Only then proceed	Risk Assessment Yes = 2; No = 0	0	0
Bleeding OF due to thrombosis	HPT(-) = 1; HPT(+) = 0 1	0	0	SIRS score $\geq$ 3 = 1	SIRS score $\geq$ 3 = 1
Platelet count ($\times$ 10^9/L)	HPT (+) = 0 HPT (-): $\leq$120 = 1 $\leq$80 = 2 $\leq$50 = 3	>100 = 0 <100 = 1 <50 = 2	>100 = 0 <100 = 1 Rising = -1 Stable = 0 Falling = 1	>120 = 0 $\geq$80 and <120 or >30% $\downarrow$ 24h = 1 <80 or >50% $\downarrow$ in 24hr = 3	>120 = 0 $\geq$80 and <120 or >30% $\downarrow$ 24h = 1 <80 or >50% $\downarrow$ in 24hr = 3
Fibrin Related Markers (FRMs)	FDPs(μg/mL): $\geq$10 = 1 $\geq$20 = 2 $\geq$40 = 3	FDP, D-dimer, SF No increase = 0 Moderate increase = 2 Strong increase = 3	Normal = 0 Raised = 1 Falling = -1 Stable = 0 Rising = 1	FDPs(mg/mL): <10 = 0 $\geq$10 = 1 $\geq$25 = 3	FDPs(mg/mL): <10 = 0 $\geq$10 = 1 $\geq$25 = 3
(Prolonged) Prothrombin time (PT)	PT ratio: $\geq$1.25 = 1 $\geq$1.67 = 2	<3 s = 0 >3 s = 1 >6 s = 2	<3 s = 0 >3 s = 1 Falling = -1 Stable = 0 Rising = 1	PT ratio: <1.2 = 0 $\geq$1.2 = 1	PT ratio: <1.2 = 0 $\geq$1.2 = 1

Scoring System	Japanese Ministry of Health and Welfare	International Society of Thrombosis and Hemostasis (ISTH) DIC score (2001)		Japanese Association for Acute Medicine (JAAM)	
				DIC score (2006)	
	(JMHW) DIC score (1988)	Overt DIC score	Non-overt DIC score	JAAM DIC score	Revised JAAM DIC score
Parameter		Parameter Value or Range = Score			
Fibrinogen level (mg/dL)	≤150 = 1	>100 = 0	Not included	<350 = 1	Not included
	≤ 100 = 2	<100 = 1		≥350 = 0	
Additional tests	No	No	Specific criteria:	No	No
			Antithrombin (AT) (Normal: -1; Low: 1) Protein-C (Normal: -1; Low: 1) TAT complex (Normal: -1; High: 1) Normal: -1 Abnormal: 1		
Diagnosis of DIC	HPT(+): ≥4	>5	≥5	≥5	≥4
	HPT(-): ≥7	<5 (indicative but not affirmative for non-overt DIC)			

Adapted from Critical Care Clinics 2012; 28(3) 373-388, Satoshi Gando: The Utility of a Diagnostic Scoring System for Disseminated Intravascular Coagulation., Copyright (2012), with permission from Elsevier.

Abbreviations: OF, organ failure; HPT, hematopoietic tumor; FDP, fibrin(ogen) degradation product; SF, soluble fibrin; TAT complex, Thrombin antithrombin complex; APS, antiphospholipid syndrome; EDTA, ethylenediaminetetraacetic acid; HELLP, hemolysis, elevated liver enzymes, and low platelet; HIT, heparin-induced thrombocytopenia; HPS, hemophagocytic syndrome; HUS, hemolytic uremic syndrome; ITP, idiopathic thrombocytopenic purpura; $PaCO_2$ partial pressure of carbon dioxide, arterial; TTP, thrombotic thrombocytopenic purpura.

1. JMHW DIC score: Differentiates between patients with [HPT (+)] and without [HPT (-)] hematopoietic malignancies.

2. ISTH ''Overt'' DIC score: (1) Mandatory risk assessment (2) An overall cumulative score of >5 is compatible with overt DIC. (3) A score <5 may be indicative (but not affirmative) of non-overt DIC.

3. ISTH ''non-overt'' DIC: (1) Includes scoring for changing values of routine tests over time; (2) Score of ≥5 is considered as permitting the diagnosis of non-overt DIC [Reference 4, 26, 34].

4. For both ISTH scoring systems: (1) PT=seconds above upper limit of reference range; (2) Degree of elevation in fibrin-related markers to be locally defined.

5. JAAM DIC score: (1) Both "underlying disease associated with DIC" and those to be "carefully ruled out" to be taken into account; (2) For presence of ≥3 SIRS criteria add 1 point to score; (2) DIC is diagnosed when the cumulative score is ≥5 in the JAAM DIC score and ≥4 in revised JAAM score.

6. Clinical conditions that may be associated with ISTH overt DIC score:
   a. Sepsis/severe infection (any microorganism);
   b. Trauma (e.g., Polytrauma/Neurotrauma/ Fat embolism)
   c. Organ dysfunction (e.g., severe pancreatitis)
   d. Malignancy (Solid tumors, Myeloproliferative/Lymphoproliferative malignancies)
   e. Obstetric calamities (Amniotic fluid embolism/Abruptio placentae)
   f. Vascular abnormalities (Kasabach-Meritt syndrome/Large vascular aneurysms)
   g. Severe hepatic failure
   h. Severe toxic or immunologic reactions (Snakebite/Recreational drugs/Transfusion reactions/Transplant rejection).

7. Clinical conditions that may be associated with DIC in JAAM DIC score:
   a. Sepsis/severe infection (any microorganism)
   b. Trauma /burn/surgery
   c. Malignancy (except bone marrow suppression)
   d. Obstetric calamities
   e. Vascular abnormalities (Large vascular aneurysms/Giant hemangioma/Vasculitis)
   f. Conditions that may be associated with SIRS (Organ destruction -e.g., severe pancreatitis/Severe hepatic failure/Ischemia/ hypoxia/shock/ Heat stroke/malignant syndrome/Fat embolism/ Rhabdomyolysis)

g. Other.
8. Clinical conditions that should be carefully ruled out in JAAM DIC score:
    a. Thrombocytopenia
        i. Dilution and abnormal distribution (Massive blood loss and transfusion, massive infusion
        ii. Increased platelet destruction (ITP, TTP/HUS, HIT drugs, viral infection, alloimmune destruction, APS, HELLP, extracorporeal circulation)
        iii. Decreased platelet production (Viral infection, drugs, radiation, nutritional deficiency (vitamin B12, folic acid), disorders of hematopoiesis, liver disease, HPS)
        iv. Spurious decrease (EDTA-dependent agglutinins, insufficient anticoagulation of blood samples)
        v. Other (Hypothermia, artificial devices in the vessel)
    b. Prolonged prothrombin time (Anticoagulation therapy, anticoagulants in blood samples, vitamin K deficiency, liver cirrhosis, massive blood loss and transfusion)
    c. Elevated FDP (Thrombosis, hemostasis and wound healing, hematoma, pleural effusion, ascites, anticoagulant in blood samples, antifibrinolytic therapy)
    d. Other.
9. SIRS, Systemic Inflammatory response syndrome: (1) Temperature $>38^{\circ}C$ or $<36^{\circ}C$ (2) Heart rate >90beats/min (3) Respiratory rate >20 breaths/min or $PaCO_2<32$ torr (<4.3 kPa) (4) White blood cell >12000 cells/mm^3, or 10% immature (band) forms.

Table 2. Brief Summary of the Advantages and Limitations of the DIC scores

DIC Score	Advantages	Limitations
Japanese Ministry of Health and Welfare **(JMHW)** DIC score	• More applicable to hematologiocal malignancies • Weightage points given to the underlying disease • Predicts outcome in leukemia • High specificity in hematological malignancies	• Absence of prospective validation studies in non-hematological malignancies [57] • Has limited utility for other etiologies of DIC • Has moderate sensitivity
International Society of Thrombosis and Hemostasis **(ISTH)** DIC score	• Utility in critical care settings both in adults and children [25, 48] • More applicable to both infective and non-infective etiologies of DIC [42, 43] • Differentiation between overt and non-overt DIC, offers opportunity to treat at the non-overt DIC stage when it may be more effective than overt DIC [4, 44, 45] • Use of multiple FRMs [FDP, D-dimer, SF], increases its potential applicability • Has higher specificity than other scores	• Restrictive usage mandates prior risk assessment before further evaluation for overt-DIC • Abscence of prospective validation studies in malignancies [57] • Diagnosis of non-overt DIC requires hemoststic markers, whose availability and applicability are not universal • Subjective criteria used for FDP and SF • Despite negligible impact of fibrinogen on diagnostic accuracy [25, 48] it continues to be used

Japanese Association for Acute Medicine (**JAAM**) DIC score	• More applicable in critical care settings [20, 58] • Easy applicability as neither weightage to underlying disease nor mandatory risk assessment required • The inclusion of SIRS and rate of decline of platelets [3, 4, 36, 46, 47] has increased its sensitivity and thus helps better select patients for early treatment of DIC • Fibrinogen excluded as it did not affect it's diagnostic accuracy [20] • Diagnoses DIC earlier than the other two scores and also shows progression to ISTH overt DIC [20, 35, 58] • Diagnoses all ISTH overt DIC cases and also those not diagnosed by ISTH overt DIC score[20, 58] • Correlation seen with JMWH and ISTH scores in septic patients [20, 43]	• Absence of data on its utility in children • Absence of prospective validation studies in malignancies [57] • Poor discriminatory power between survivors and non-survivors amongst DIC patients at lower APACHE II scores [54, 55, 56] • Has moderate specificity [20]

Abbreviations: SIRS, systemic inflammatory response syndrome; FRMs, fibrin related markers; FDP, fibrin(ogen) degradation product; SF, soluble fibrin;

but also most accurate score is not yet finished. Serial trends of the scores may further add to their diagnostic and prognostic efficacy. Inclusion of existing and upcoming hemostatic molecular markers within these DIC scoring systems may further enhance their effectiveness.

Acknowledgement

I wish to acknowledge Satisho Gando and Elsevier for insights gained about DIC scores from their publication: Gando S. The utility of a diagnostic scoring system for disseminated intravascular coagulation. *Crit Care Clin.* 2012 Jul;28(3):373-88.

References

[1]   Levi, M. Disseminated intravascular coagulation. *Crit. Care Med.* 2007; 35:2191–5.

[2]   Levi, M. Disseminated intravascular coagulation: What's new? *Crit. Care Clin.* 2005;21:449–67.

[3]   Levi, M., Ten Cate, H. Disseminated intravascular coagulation. *N Engl. J. Med.* 1999;341:586–92.

[4]   Taylor, Jr F. B., Toh, C. H., Hoot, W. K., et al. Toward definition, clinical and laboratory criteria, and a scoring system for disseminated intravascular coagulation. *Thromb. Haemost.* 2001; 86:1327–30.

[5]   Esmon, C. T., Fukudome, K., Mather, T., et al. Inflammation, sepsis, and coagulation. *Hematologica* 1999;84:254–9.

[6]   Jesmin, S., Wada, T., Gando, S., et al. The dynamics of angiogenic factors and their soluble receptors in relation to organ dysfunction in disseminated intravascular coagulation associated with sepsis. *Inflammation.* 2013;36(1):186-96.

[7]   Wada, T., Jesmin, S., Gando, S., et al. Using angiogenic factors and their soluble receptors to predict organ dysfunction in patients with disseminated intravascular coagulation associated with severe trauma. *Crit. Care.* 2012;16(2):R63.

[8]   Eskici, Z. M., Açıkgöz, Ş., Pişkin, N., et al. High mobility group B1 levels in sepsis and Disseminated Intravascular Coagulation. *Acta Biochim. Pol.* 2012;59(4):561-6.

[9]   Wada, H., Wakita, Y., Nakase, T., et al. Outcome prediction of disseminated intravascular coagulation in relation to the score when treatment was begun. *Thromb. Haemost.* 1995;74:848–52.

[10]   Dhainaut, J. F., Yan, S. B., Joyce, D. E., et al. Treatment effects of drotrecogin alfa (activated) in patients with severe sepsis with or without overt disseminated intravascular coagulation. *J. Thromb. Haemost.* 2004;2: 1924–33.

[11]   Bick, R. Disseminated intravascular coagulation, old disease, new hope. *BMJ* 2003;327: 974-7.

[12]   Levi, M., Toh, C. H., Thachil, J., et al. Guidelines for diagnosis and management of disseminated intravascular coagulation. British Committee for Standards in Hematology. *Br. J. Haematol.* 2009;145:24-33.

[13]   Toh, C. H.: Laboratory testing in disseminated intravascular coagulation. *Semin. Thromb. Haemost.* 2001; 27:653–656].

[14]   Prisco, D., Paniccia, R., Boneichi, F., et al. Evaluation of new methods for the selective measurement of fibrin and fibriniogen degradation products. *Thromb. Res.* 1989;56 :547-51.

[15]   Shorr, A. F., Trotta, R. F., Alkins, S. A., et al. D-dimer assay predicts mortality in critically ill patients without disseminated intravascular coagulation or venous thromboembolic disease. *Intensive Care Med.* 1999;25:207-10.

[16]   Wada, H., Asakura, H., Okamoto, K., et al. Expert consensus for the treatment of disseminated intravascular coagulation in Japan. *Thromb. Res.* 2010;125:6–11.

[17]   Di Nisio, M., Baudo, F., Cosmi, B., et al. Diagnosis and treatment of disseminated intravascular coagulation: Guidelines of the Italian Society for Haemostasis and Thrombosis (SISET). *Thrombo. Res.* 2012; 129 (5): e177-e84.

[18]   Wada, H., Gabazza, E. C., Asakura, H., et al. Comparison of diagnostic criteria for disseminated intravascular coagulation (DIC): Diagnostic criteria of the international society of thrombosis and haemostasis (ISTH) and of the Japanese Ministry of Health and Welfare for overt DIC. *Am. J. Hematol.* 2003;74:17–22.

[19]   Kobayashi, N., Maekawa, T., Takeda, M., et al. Criteria for diagnosis of DIC based on the analysis of clinical and laboratory findings in 345 DIC patients collected by the Research Committee on DIC in Japan. *Bibl. Haematol.* 1987;49:848–52.

[20] Gando, S., Iba, T., Eguchi, Y., et al. A multicenter, prospective validation of disseminated intravascular coagulation diagnostic criteria for critically ill patients: comparing current criteria. *Crit. Care Med.* 2006;34: 625–31.

[21] Kawasugi, K., Wada, H., Hatada, T., et al. Japanese Society of Thrombosis Hemostasis/DIC subcommittee. Prospective evaluation of hemostatic abnormalities in overt DIC due to various underlying diseases. *Thromb. Res.* 2011; 128:186-90.

[22] Wada, H., thachi, J., Di Nisio, et al. Guidance for diagnosis and treatment of disseminated intravascular coagulation from harmonization of the recommendations from three guidelines. *J. Thromb. Haemost.* 2013;11:761-7.

[23] Kienast, J., Juers, M., Wiedermann, C. J., et al. Treatment effects of high dose antithrombin without concomittant heparin in patients with severe sepsis with or without disseminated intravascular coagulation. *J. Thromb. Haemost.* 2006;4;90-7.

[24] Angstwurm, M. W., Dempfle, C. E., Spannagl, M. New disseminated intravascular coagulation score: a useful tool to predict mortality in comparison with Acute Physiology and Chronic Health Evaluation II and Logistic organ Dysfunction scores. *Crit. Care Med.* 2006;34:327-33.

[25] Bakhtiari, K., Meijers, J. C., de Jonge, E., et al. Prospective validation of the International Society of Thrombosis and Haemostasis scoring system for disseminated intravascular coagulation. *Crit. Care Med.* 2004;32: 2416–21.

[26] Toh, C. H., Hoots, W. K. The scoring system of the Scientific and Standardisation Committee on Disseminated Intravascular Coagulation of the International Society on Thrombosis and Haemostasis: A 5-year overview. *J. Thromb. Haemost.* 2007;5:604–606.

[27] Hayakawa, M., Gando, S., Hoshino, H. A prospective comparison of new Japanese criteria for disseminated intravascular coagulation: New Japanese criteria versus ISTH criteria. *Clin. Appl. Thromb. Hemost.* 2007;13:172–181.

[28] Egi, M., Morimatsu, H., Wiedermann, C. J., et al. Non-overt disseminated intravascular coagulation scoring for critically ill patients: The impact of antithrombin levels. *Thromb. Haemost.* 2009;101:696–705.

[29] Toh, C. H., Downey, C. Performance and prognostic importance of a new clinical and laboratory scoring system for identifying non-overt

disseminated intravascular coagulation. *Blood Coagul. Fibrinolysis* 2005;16:69–74.

[30] Wada, H., Gabazza, E. C., Nakasaki, T., et al. Diagnosis of disseminated intravascular coagulation by hemostatic molecular markers. *Semin. Thromb. Hemost.* 2000;26:17–22.

[31] Wada, H., Sakuragawa, N., Shiku, H. Hemostatic molecular markers before onset of disseminated intravascular coagulation in leukemic patients. *Semin. Thromb. Hemost.* 1998;24:293–297.

[32] Dempfle, C. E. Comparing DIC scores: not an easy task indeed. *Throm. Res.* 2009;124:651-2.

[33] Oh, D., Jang, M. J., Lee, S. J., et al. Evaluation of modified non-overt DIC criteria on the prediction of poor outcome in patients with sepsis. *Thromb. Res.* 2010;126(1):18-23.

[34] Wada, H., Hatada, T., Okamoto, K., et al. Japanese Society of Thrombosis Hemostasis/DIC subcommittee. Modified non-overt DIC diagnostic criteria predict the early phase of overt-DIC. *Am. J. Hematol.* 2010;85(9):691-4.

[35] Gando, S., Saitoh, D., Ogura, H., et al. Natural history of disseminted intravascular coagulation diagnosed based on newly established diagnostic criteria for critically ill patients: results of a multicenter, prospective survey. *Crit. Care Med.* 2008;36:145-50.

[36] Esmon, C. T.: Inflammation and thrombosis. *J. Thromb. Haemost.* 2003; 1:1343–1348

[37] Sawamura, A., Hayakawa, M., Gando, S., et al. Disseminated intravascular coagulation with a fibrinolytic phenotype at an early phase of trauma predicts mortality. *Thromb. Res.* 2009;124:608–13.

[38] Sawamura, A., Hayakawa, M., Gando, S., et al. Application of the Japanese Association for Acute Medicine disseminated intravascular coagulation diagnostic criteria for patients at an early phase of trauma. *Thromb. Res.* 2009;124:706–10.

[39] Kobayashi, T., Terao, T., Maki, M., et al. Diagnosis of management of acute obstetrical DIC. *Semin. Thromb. Hemost.* 2001;27:161-7.

[40] Henzan, N., Gando, S., Uegaki, S., et al. Disseminated intravascular coagulation (DIC) in acute leukemia using newly developed DIC diagnostic criteria for critically ill patients. *JJAAM* 2007; 18:793-802.

[41] Gando, S., Saitoh, D., Ogura, H., et al. Disseminated intravascular coagulation (DIC) diagnosed based on the Japanese Association for Acute Medicine criteria is a dependent continuum to overt DIC in patients with sepsis. *Throm. Res.* 2009;123:715-8.

[42] Hatada, T., Wada, H., Nobori, T., et al. Plasma concentrations and importance and importance of high mobility group box protein in the prognosis of organ failure in patients with disseminated intra vascular coagulation. *Throm. Haemost.* 2005;94:975-9.

[43] Gando, S., Wada, H., Asakura, H., et al. Evaluation of new Japanese diagnostic criteria for disseminated intravascular coagulation in critically ill patients. *Clin. Appl. Thromb. Hemost.* 2005;11:71-6.

[44] Taylor, F. B., Kinasewiz, G. T. The diagnosis and management of disseminated intravascular coagulation. *Current Hematol. Rep.* 2002;1: 34-40.

[45] Hoots, W. K. Non-overt disseminated intravascular coagulation: definition and pathophysiological implications. *Blood Rev.* 2002;16 (Suppl. 1): S3-9.

[46] Range-Frausto, M. S., Pittet, D., Costigan, M., et al.: The natural history of the systemic inflammatory response syndrome (SIRS): A prospective study. *JAMA* 1995; 273:117–123

[47] Akca, S., Haji-Michael, P., de Mendonça, A., et al.: Time course of platelet counts in critically ill patients. *Crit. Care Med.* 2002; 30:753–756

[48] Soundar, E. P., Jariwala, P., Nguyen, T. C., et al. Evaluation of the international society on thrombosis and haemostasis and institutional diagnostic criteria of disseminated intravascular coagulation in pediatric patients. *Am. J. Clin. Pathol.* 2013;139(6):812-6.

[49] Wada, H., Wakita, Y., Nakase, T., et al. Mie DIC Study Group. Outcome of disseminted intravascular coagulation in relation to the score when treatment was begun. *Thromb. Haemost.* 1995;74:848-52.

[50] Khemani, R. G., Bart, R. D., Alonzo, T. A., et al. Disseminated intravascular coagulation score is associated with mortality for children with shock. *Intensive Care Med.* 2009;35(2):327-33.

[51] Takemitsu, T., Wada, H., Hatada, T., et al. Prospective evaluation of three different diagnostic criteria for disseminted intravascular coagulation. *Thromb. Haemost.* 2011;105:40-4.

[52] Bick, R. Disseminted intravascular coagulation: Objective clinical and laboratory diagnosis, treatment, and assessment of therapeutic response. *Semin. Thromb. Hemost.* 1996;22:69-88.

[53] Toh, C. H., Dennis, M. Disseminted intravascular coagulation, old disease new hope. *BMJ* 2003;327:974-7.

[54] Singh, R. K., Baronia, A. K., Sahoo, J. N., et al. Prospective comparison of new Japanese Association for Acute medicine (JAAM) DIC and

International Society of Thrombosis and Hemostasis (ISTH) DIC score in critically ill septic patients. *Throm. Res.* 2012;129(4);e119-25.

[55] Iwai, K., Uchino, S., Endo, A., et al. Prospective external validation of the new scoring system for disseminated intravascular coagulation by Japanese Association for Acute medicine (JAAM). *Thromb. Res.* 2010; 126:217-21.

[56] Sivula, M., Tallgren, M., Pettila, V. Modified scorer for disseminated intravascular coagulation in the critically ill. *Intensive Care Med.* 2005; 31:1209-14.

[57] Gando S. The utility of a diagnostic scoring system for disseminated intravascular coagulation. Crit Care Clin. 2012 Jul;28(3):373-88.

[58] Gando S, Saitoh D, Ogura H, Fujishima S., et al. A multicenter, prospective validation study of the Japanese Association for Acute Medicine disseminated intravascular coagulation scoring system in patients with severe sepsis. Critical Care 2013, 17:R111.

In: Disseminated Intravascular Coagulation (DIC)   ISBN: 978-1-62948-323-8
Editor: Balwinder Singh   © 2014 Nova Science Publishers, Inc.

Chapter V

Outcome of Critically Ill Patients with Disseminated Intravascular Coagulation in a Tertiary Care Center

Balwinder Singh MD,[1,] Rabe' Elias Alhurani MBBS[1] and Pablo Moreno Franco MD[2]*

[1]Department of Medicine, Division of Pulmonary and
Critical Care Medicine, Mayo Clinic, Rochester, MN, US
[2]Department of Medicine, Division of Transplant
Critical Care Service, Mayo Clinic, Jacksonville, Florida, US

Abstract

Background: We aimed to determine the prognostic factors influencing the hospital mortality of the critically ill patients with disseminated intravascular coagulation (DIC).

Method: We conducted a population-based historical cohort study evaluating consecutively admitted adult overt DIC patients from Olmsted County at the Mayo Clinic ICUs, from 2004-2010. DIC was diagnosed

* Corresponding author: Balwinder Singh, MD; E-mail:singh.balwinder@alumni.mayo.edu.

according to the International Society on Thrombosis and Hemostasis overt DIC algorithm.

The prognostic factors included were patient's demographics, comorbidities, severity of illness scores and risk factors for DIC. Multivariate logistic regression analysis was used to identify the independent predictors associated with hospital death.

Results: A total of 154 patients met the overt DIC criteria, 61 females (40%), median age of 63 years (IQR 52-76) and 128 (83%) were Caucasians. The hospital mortality was 50.6 %. On univariate analysis, age, severe sepsis, septic shock, acute respiratory failure (ARF), heparin use, history of congestive heart failure (CHF) and diabetes with organ damage were associated with hospital mortality. In the multivariate logistic regression analysis, septic shock (Odds ratio [OR] 2.27, 95% confidence interval [CI] 1.12 - 4.66), ARF (OR 2.28, 95% CI 1.15 - 4.58) and history of CHF (OR 3.57, 95% CI 1.26 - 11.8) were identified as the independent predictors for hospital mortality in critically ill DIC patients.

Conclusion: ARF, Septic shock and history of CHF are independent predictors for hospital mortality in DIC patients. Early diagnosis, better management of ARF and Septic shock patients, along with history of CHF, may contribute better outcomes among DIC patients in the ICUs.

Keywords: Disseminated Intravascular Coagulation; Outcomes; Septic shock, acute respiratory failure; Predictors; Hospital mortality

Introduction

Disseminated intravascular coagulation (DIC) is a coagulation disorder characterized by systemic activation of widespread thrombosis, contributing to intravascular fibrin generation and clot formation, resulting in inadequate blood supply to organs leading to organ failure [1].

In 2001, the International Society on Thrombosis and Hemostasis (ISTH) Scientific Subcommittee on DIC proposed a scoring system to diagnose DIC and an algorithm to further sub-divide DIC into overt and non-overt DIC [2], based on the presence or absence of underlying predisposing conditions. Patients admitted to the intensive care units (ICU) are at higher risk for developing DIC [1, 3]. DIC is a devastating syndrome with major morbidity and mortality in the critically ill patients [1, 3-6].

Therefore, it is essential to understand and determine the prognosis of critically ill patients with DIC who require ICU admission. Previous studies have identified the severity of illness [7] and sepsis [8] as poor prognostic factors of DIC.

However, specific prognostic features including demographics, comorbidities, and presence of predisposing factors such as septic shock, acute lung injury (ALI), acute respiratory failure (ARF) and the effects of treatment therapies have not been systematically studied.

Early diagnosis and accurate prognosis are important in improving the outcomes of patients with DIC [6]. In a recently published study, we estimated that the incidence of DIC in critically ill patients is decreasing, however, the mortality rate is still very high [6]. Therefore, we aimed to identify the prognostic factors predicting the hospital mortality of the critically ill patients with overt DIC.

Some of the study findings have been previously reported in the form of an abstract [9].

Methods

Population: We conducted a population-based historical cohort study of adult (≥18 years) Olmsted County residents, diagnosed with overt DIC, who were admitted to the Mayo Clinic ICUs in Rochester, MN, from January 1, 2004 to December 31, 2010 [6]. The Mayo Clinic Institutional Review Board approved the study. The Mayo Clinic in Rochester, MN is an academic medical center comprising two hospitals - Rochester Methodist Hospital and Saint Mary's Hospital, with 1900 hospital and 164 adult ICU patient beds [3]. The Mayo Clinic hospitals, together with Olmsted Medical center, administer > 95% of the primary, secondary and tertiary care provided to the Olmsted county population. [10] This provides us an excellent opportunity to identify the characteristics of all the cases in Olmsted County with complete detail.

Case identification: We used the ISTH overt DIC algorithm to identify overt DIC patients, with a cumulative score of 5 or above as the diagnostic criteria, using platelet counts, prothrombin time, fibrinogen level, and D-Dimer level as the fibrin related marker [2, 6]. D-dimer level >1 μg/mL was considered moderate increase and >4 μg/mL as severe increase, as per the recommendations of 49th SSC meeting of ISTH [5, 11]. Patients who denied research authorization, those diagnosed with heparin induced thrombo-cytopenia, thrombotic thrombocytopenic purpura, Child Pugh class C or any known congenital coagulation disorders were excluded from the study. The electronic medical records (EMR) of all the patients meeting overt DIC criteria were comprehensively reviewed by physician investigators to identify and confirm the DIC diagnosis and the predisposing conditions.

The inter-reviewer agreement between the two physician investigators to diagnose DIC and the predisposing conditions was excellent [6]. Figure 1 provides the details for the ascertainment of DIC cases.

Data extraction: A standardized protocol was used for the extraction of data from the institutional databases and EMR, wherein trained research coordinators and critical care research fellows extracted the data from the EMR.

Patient's demographics, baseline characteristics, severity of illness [using Acute Physiology and Chronic Health Evaluation (APACHE) III score], organ failure [using Sequential Organ Failure Assessment score (SOFA) score] were extracted from the ICU database which had been validated previously [12]. The Charlson index was used to assess the comorbidity status, which was extracted using reliable automated digital algorithms [13, 14].

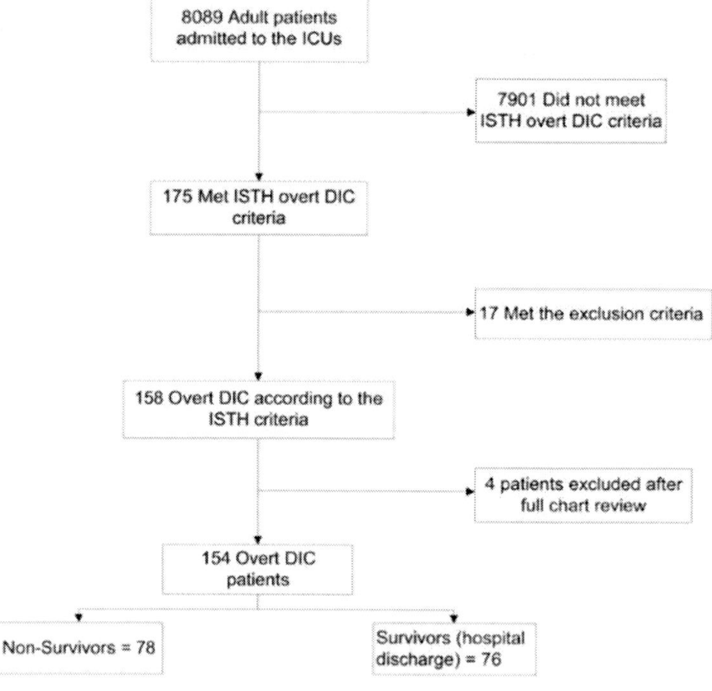

Figure 1. The study flow diagram for the ascertainment of DIC cases.

The prognostic factors included were patient's demographics (age, sex, race) baseline comorbidities (respiratory, cardiac, hepatic, renal, lympho-reticular and malignancy), APACHE III, Charlson and SOFA scores and predictors of DIC. The prognostic factors were defined according to the standardized criteria (Severe sepsis and septic shock [15, 16], shock [17], ALI [18], acute liver failure [19], ARF [20], acute kidney injury(AKI) [21]). The primary outcome of the patients with DIC was hospital mortality. The death date of each patient was identified from the EMR and death registration record of Minnesota in the event of out-of-hospital deaths.

Statistical Analysis

Continuous variables are reported as mean [standard deviation (SD)], median [interquartile range (IQR)] and categorical variables as counts and percentages. The unpaired Student's-t test and Mann-Whitney U test are used to compare continuous variables with normal distribution and for skewed distribution respectively. We used chi-square and Fisher's exact test for the comparison of categorical variables, depending on the number of elements in each cell. We used a univariate and stepwise multiple logistic regression model to estimate the associations between demographics, comorbidities, APACHE III, Charlson and SOFA scores, prognostic factors for DIC, and hospital mortality as the outcome, and was presented as odds ratios (ORs) with 95% CIs. We introduced the significant variables on univariate analysis with P values < 0.1 into a multivariate logistic regression model. Stepwise backward and forward logistic regression model were used, where in one non-significant variable was removed at a time. P-values <0.05 were considered statistically significant for multivariate analysis. Kaplan–Meier analysis was performed to assess the short term (hospital) mortality and compared using Log-Rank test. JMP 9.0.1 computer software (SAS Institute, Cary, NC) was used for the analysis.

Results

A total of 154 patients met the inclusion criteria for DIC from a cohort of 8089 adult patients admitted to the ICUs (Figure 1). In the study cohort, 61 (40%) were females, median age of 63 years (IQR 52-76) and 128 (83%) were

Caucasians. The median APACHE III score, Charlson index and SOFA scores on day one were 97 (IQR, 68 - 120), 3 (IQR, 1- 5) and 10 (IQR, 6 - 13) respectively. Seventy eight (50.6%) patients diagnosed with DIC died during the hospitalization. The median time to hospital death after DIC onset was 5 days (IQR 1-10 days).

While the survivors were younger (60 vs. 67, p = 0.042), the severity of illness was similar between the survivors and non-survivors (median APACHE III score 93 vs. 102, p = 0.098). The overall comorbidity status measured by Charlson comorbidity score was similar among the survivors and non-survivors, however, the comorbidities significantly associated with mortality were congestive heart failure (CHF), and diabetes with complications or end-organ damage (Table 1). The differences in the baseline characteristics, risk factors, treatment and outcomes between the DIC survivors and non-survivors are shown in table 1. There were 92 severe sepsis cases (59.7%), 59 septic shock cases (38.3%) and 68 ARF cases (44.2%). The survivors with DIC had less severe sepsis (50 % vs. 69%, p = 0.015), septic shock (26% vs. 50%, p = 0.003), and ARF cases (33% vs. 55%, p = 0.006) as compared to non-survivors. There was no difference in mortality between the DIC cases with other critical care syndromes of ARDS and AKI.

DIC treatment including the use of heparin alone, heparin with fresh frozen plasma (FFP) and platelets, FFP/platelets alone, cryoprecipitate with FFP and platelets, and activated protein-C (APC) [22] is summarized in Table 1. Compared to non-survivor DIC patients, survivors with DIC were more often prescribed heparin (29% vs. 16%; p = 0.04). There was no difference in the use of other therapies between the DIC patients who survived and who did not survive (Table 1). On subset analysis, we observed that the patients initiated on APC had a higher median SOFA score (14; IQR 8-15) as compared to the rest of DIC patients (median SOFA score of 10; IQR 6-12) (not shown in the tables). The median (IQR) lengths of ICU and hospital stays were 2.9 days (1.2–7.1) and 12.0 days (6.2-24.8), respectively. There was no significant difference between the ICU and hospital length of stays between the survivors and non-survivors of DIC.

On univariate analysis, age, shock (any kind), severe sepsis, septic shock, ARF, heparin use, history of CHF and diabetes with organ damage were associated with hospital mortality. In the multivariate logistic regression analysis, Septic shock (Odds ratio [OR] 2.27, 95% confidence interval [CI] 1.12 - 4.66), ARF (OR 2.28, 95% CI 1.15 - 4.58) and history of CHF (OR 3.57, 95% CI 1.26 - 11.82) were identified as the independent predictors associated with in-hospital death (Table 2).

Table 1. Differences in baseline characteristics, risk factors, medications, and outcomes between hospital survivors and non-survivors (among DIC patients)

Variable	Survivors (n = 76)	Non-survivors (n = 78)	p-value
Demographics			
Age years, median (IQR)	60 (50.6 - 70.4)	67 (54.0 - 77.8)	0.04
Sex, Female (%)	27 (36)	34 (44)	0.31
Race, Caucasian (%)	63 (83)	65 (83)	0.94
APACHE III score, median (IQR)	93 (60 - 112)	102 (71 - 127)	0.10
SOFA score on day one, median (IQR)	10 (6 - 13)	10 (7 - 12)	0.92
Charlson score, median (IQR)	3 (1 - 5)	4 (2 - 5)	0.24
DIC time from admission, median (IQR)	79 (19 - 149)	54 (14 - 199)	0.12
Comorbidities, N (%)			
Cancer	16 (21)	19 (24)	0.62
Congestive heart failure	5 (7)	16 (21)	0.01
Diabetes with organ damage	1 (1)	9 (12)	0.01
Cirrhosis	10 (14)	17 (22)	0.16
Leukemia	3 (4)	5 (6)	1.00
Lymphoma	6 (8)	9 (12)	0.45
Medications, N (%)			
Heparin	22 (29)	12 (16)	0.04
Heparin + Platelets/FFP	27 (35)	27 (35)	0.91
Platelets/FFP	11 (14)	20 (26)	0.08
APC	2 (3)	6 (8)	0.28
Others	14 (18)	13 (17)	0.78
Risk factors, N (%)			
Severe Sepsis	38 (50)	54 (69)	0.02
Septic Shock	20 (26)	39 (50)	0.003
Pneumonia	13 (17)	18 (23)	0.35
Acute respiratory failure	25 (33)	43 (55)	0.005
Acute lung injury	20 (26)	32 (41)	0.05
Acute kidney injury	36 (47)	42 (54)	0.42
Acute liver failure	6 (8)	5 (6)	0.72
High risk surgery	12 (16)	14 (18)	0.72
Trauma	2 (3)	3 (4)	1.00
Outcomes			

Table 1. (Continued)

Variable	Survivors (n = 76)	Non-survivors (n = 78)	p-value
Outcomes			
ICU length of stay, d, median (IQR)	3.0 (1.5 - 6.3)	2.8 (1.1 - 8.3)	0.26
Hospital length of stay, d, median (IQR)	14.7 (8.5 - 25.8)	8.9 (2.8 - 23.2)	0.32
Invasive mechanical ventilation (IMV) used, n (%)	53 (70)	60 (77)	0.31
Non-invasive mechanical ventilation used, n (%)	14 (18)	17 (22)	0.60
IMV days, median (IQR)	0.6 (0 - 2.8)	0.9 (0 - 6.7)	0.31
Duration of ventilation, median (IQR)	0.7 (0 – 3.0)	1.2 (0.2 - 7.6)	0.27

APACHE = Acute Physiology and Chronic Health Evaluation; APC= activated protein C; DIC=disseminated intravascular coagulation; IQR=interquartile range; SOFA= Sequential Organ Failure Assessment score.

Figure 2 (A, B and C) shows the survival curves for septic shock, ARF and patients with history of CHF, respectively. Even on including the APACHE III scores in the model, all the three predictors remained significant, with OR for septic shock, ARF and CHF (comorbidity) as 2.16, 2.24 and 3.46 respectively (Table 3).

Discussion

Disseminated intravascular coagulation is a devastating syndrome with major morbidity and mortality in the critically ill patients [1, 3, 6]. In this study, we observed that the presence of septic shock, ARF and history of CHF are independent predictors of the hospital mortality in DIC patients. In contrast to previous studies, we did not find severity of illness (APACHE score) and age as independent predictors of death [7, 23]. Although age was associated with death on univariate analysis, it was not significant on multivariable analysis. The probable reason for absence of APACHE III as a mortality predictor could be due to overall high severity of illness in our study cohort. However, even after including the APACHE III score in the model, septic shock, CHF and ARF remained as significant predictors of hospital mortality. Thus, confirming their substantial effect on the mortality among the DIC patients.

Table 2. Univariate and multivariate models for hospital mortality among DIC patients

Variables	Univariate analysis			Multivariate analysis		
	Odds Ratio	95% CI	p- value	Odds Ratio	95% CI	p- value
Acute kidney injury	1.30	0.69 - 2.45	0.42			
Acute liver failure	0.80	0.22 - 2.77	0.72			
Acute lung injury	1.95	0.99 -3.89	0.05			
Acute respiratory failure	2.51	1.31 - 4.87	0.005[*]	2.28	1.15-4.58	0.019
Age	1.02	1.00 - 1.04	0.04[*]			
APACHE III score	1.01	0.999 - 1.02	0.10			
Atrial fibrillation	0.57	0.11 - 2.40	0.44			
Cancer	1.21	0.57 - 2.60	0.62			
Charlson	1.07	0.96 - 1.2	0.24			
Cirrhosis	1.84	0.79 - 4.46	0.16			
Congestive heart failure	3.66	1.35– 11.72	0.01[*]	3.57	1.26-1.82	0.016
COPD	0.65	0.26 - 1.56	0.34			
Diabetes with organ damage	9.78	1.77-182.71	0.01[*]			
DIC time from admission	1.00	0.999- .002	0.10			
Only Heparin	0.45	0.20 - 0.97	0.04[*]			
Heparin use[**]	0.55	0.29 - 1.05	0.07			
High risk surgery	1.17	0.50 - 2.75	0.72			
Hospital LOS	0.99	0.98 - 1.01	0.32			
ICU LOS	1.02	0.99 - 1.06	0.24			
IMV days	1.02	0.99 - 1.06	0.30			
Invasive Ventilation use	1.45	0.70 - 3.00	0.31			
Pneumonia	1.45	0.66 - 3.28	0.35			
Post operative	0.71	0.22 - 2.14	0.54			
Renal disease	1.03	0.50 - 2.11	0.93			
Severe Sepsis	2.25	1.18 - 4.39	0.01[*]			
Septic Shock	2.80	1.44 - 5.58	0.002[*]	2.27	1.22-4.66	0.024
Sex	1.40	0.73 - 2.70	0.31			
Shock	2.32	1.23 - 4.47	0.01[*]			
SOFA day one	1.01	0.92- 1.10	0.91			
Trauma	1.48	0.24-11.48	0.67			
Ventilation days	1.02	0.99 - 1.06	0.25			

[*]statistically significant.

[**]it includes the entire patient with Heparin use (heparin and/or heparin + platelets/ FFP).

Table 3. Multivariate model for hospital mortality including the APACHE III score

Multivariate analysis			
Risk factors	Odds Ratio	95% CI	P - value
APACHE III score	1.01	0.995 – 1.02	0.35
Acute respiratory failure	2.24	1.13 - 4.53	0.02
Congestive heart failure	3.46	1.22 - 11.47	0.02
Septic Shock	2.16	1.06 - 4.47	0.03

One of the important finding of our study, is the presence of CHF as a strong predictor for hospital mortality. The increased risk of mortality in subjects with DIC supports the potential effects of heart failure on the platelets and coagulation system. Patients with heart failure are more likely to have activation of platelets and coagulation system [24-26], endothelial dysfunction and higher proinflammatory cytokine and adhesion molecule levels [26], which may contribute to the higher mortality. Use of heparin as a treatment therapy for overt DIC cases was significant on univariate analysis; however, it could not reach statistical significance on multivariate analysis. Only a minority of patients received the controversial activated protein-C or drotrecogin alpha (activated) [22, 27, 28]; hence, the data on the use of APC should be interpreted with extreme caution. As the sample size of patients who received APC is too small, just 5.2% of the whole cohort, they might have been chosen selectively to receive this treatment, hence there is a high probability of selection bias among these patients. On subset analysis, we observed that APC was used only for patients with higher number of organ failures, assessed by SOFA scores.

One of the reasons for low usage of APC could be due to physicians mistrust in the medicine, due to higher side-effects and variable results in the studies [22, 27, 29, 30]. However, in our study, we did not observe any statistical benefit for the survival among DIC patients who were initiated on the APC therapy.

In severe sepsis and septic shock, the activation of the coagulation cascade and obstruction of microvasculature is instrumental" [31]. Tissue factor and thrombin participate in causing the post-traumatic SIRS and DIC as a frequent complication of SIRS in such patients [32]. Early microcirculatory perfusion indices in severe sepsis and septic shock are more markedly impaired in non-survivor compared with survivors and with increasing severity of global cardiovascular dysfunction.

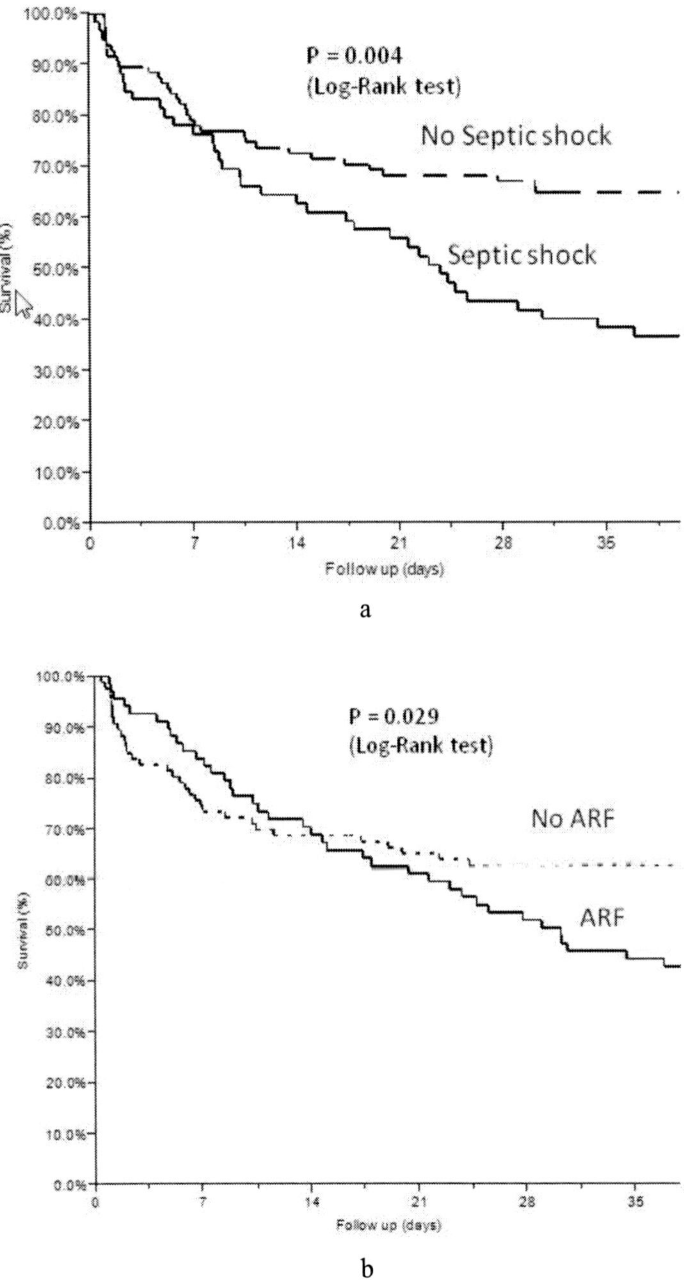

a

b

Figure 2. (Continued).

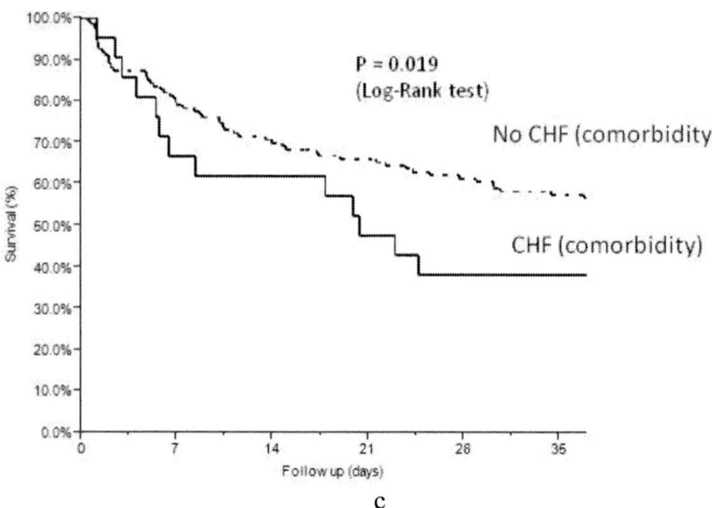

ARF=acute respiratory failure, CHF=congestive heart failure; DIC=disseminated intravascular coagulation.

Figure 2. Kaplan-Meier survival curves for A) septic shock, B) acute respiratory failure and C) congestive heart failure (comorbidity) among the DIC patients.

In sepsis and shock patients, regional tissue distress caused by microcirculatory dysfunction and mitochondrial depression produces regional hypoxia and oxygen extraction deficit, which persists despite correction of systemic oxygen delivery variables [33]. Taking these perspectives into account, the relationship between DIC and sepsis seems to be that of a direct causation, perhaps even the more complicated sepsis cases would be strongly related to DIC, this would explain the increased mortality found in our study.

In ARF patients, systemic and pulmonary bacterial infections trigger fibrin deposition along septae and intravascular micro-thromboses, thus, indicating that both alveolar space and microcirculation are affected by the inflammatory challenge. The protease activated receptor activation by tissue factor initiation reaction and downstream thrombin enhances inflammation of relevance for disease progression in ALI [34]. This could be the reason for the temporal association between ARF and DIC, thus higher mortality.

Our study has certain important limitations. Firstly, due to the retrospective-nature of our study, there is a concern for confounding and unmeasured bias. We ensured various quality measures to address these issues; two reviewers independently made the diagnosis of DIC and identified predisposing factors for a subset of patients.

The agreement between two physicians for the DIC identification and ascertainment of predisposing conditions were κ = 0.93 and 0.86 respectively, mentioned elsewhere [6]. Secondly, our study was limited to adult overt DIC patients, so these findings may not be generalizable to the pediatric populations. Thirdly, patients with ISTH DIC scores <5 and non-overt DIC cases were not included in our analysis. Hence, our findings cannot be generalized to such cases. Fourthly, the study was conducted in a tertiary care center; the patient profile might be different from the other primary care centers. However, the population based nature of this study might argue against this concern. Previous studies have shown that the results from the Olmsted County could be generalizable to the Upper-Midwest population, and may provide important information which is consistent with the national data [35].

In conclusion, we identified a strong association between septic shock, ARF, presence of CHF as comorbid condition and hospital mortality in DIC patients. Thus, early diagnosis, better management of ARF and septic shock patients, along with history of CHF, may contribute to better outcomes among critically ill DIC patients in the ICUs.

References

[1]   Levi, M., Ten Cate, H. Disseminated intravascular coagulation. *N Engl. J. Med.* 1999;341:586-592.

[2]   Taylor, F. B., Jr., Toh, C. H., Hoots, W. K., et al. Towards definition, clinical and laboratory criteria, and a scoring system for disseminated intravascular coagulation. *Thromb. Haemost.* 2001;86:1327-1330.

[3]   Cartin-Ceba, R., Kojicic, M., Li, G., et al. Epidemiology of critical care syndromes, organ failures and life support interventions in a suburban US community. *Chest* 2011;140:1447–1455.

[4]   Singh, B., Gajic, O., Li, G. Incidence and Outcome of Disseminated Intravascular Coagulation (DIC) in Olmsted County, Minnesota (2004-2010)-A Population Based Cohort Study. *Am. J. Respir. Crit. Care Med.* 2012:185: A6063.

[5]   Toh, C. H., Downey, C. Performance and prognostic importance of a new clinical and laboratory scoring system for identifying non-overt disseminated intravascular coagulation. *Blood Coagul. Fibrinolysis* 2005; 16:69-74.

[6]   Singh, B., Hanson, A. C., Alhurani, R., et al. Trends in the Incidence and Outcomes of Disseminated Intravascular Coagulation in Critically Ill Patients (2004-2010) - A Population Based Study. *Chest* 2012;143:1235-1242.

[7]   Angstwurm, M. W., Dempfle, C. E., Spannagl, M. New disseminated intravascular coagulation score: A useful tool to predict mortality in comparison with Acute Physiology and Chronic Health Evaluation II and Logistic Organ Dysfunction scores. *Crit. Care Med.* 2006;34:314-320.

[8]   Kushimoto, S., Gando, S., Saitoh, D., et al. Clinical course and outcome of disseminated intravascular coagulation diagnosed by Japanese Association for Acute Medicine criteria. Comparison between sepsis and trauma. *Thromb. Haemost.* 2008;100:1099-1105.

[9]   Singh, B., Ahmed, A., Alhurani, R., et al. Outcome of Critically ill Patients With Disseminating Intravascular Coagulation: A Population-Based Study. *Chest.* 2012;142:304A-304A.

[10] Seferian, E. G., Afessa, B. Demographic and clinical variation of adult intensive care unit utilization from a geographically defined population. *Crit. Care Med.* 2006;34:2113-2119.

[11] Egi, M., Morimatsu, H., Wiedermann, C. J., et al. Non-overt disseminated intravascular coagulation scoring for critically ill patients: the impact of antithrombin levels. *Thrombosis and haemostasis* 2009; 101:696-705.

[12] Herasevich, V., Pickering, B. W., Dong, Y., et al. Informatics infrastructure for syndrome surveillance, decision support, reporting, and modeling of critical illness. *Mayo Clin. Proc.* 2010;85:247-254.

[13] Singh, B., Singh, A., Ahmed, A., et al. Derivation and validation of automated electronic search strategies to extract Charlson comorbidities from the electronic medical records. *Mayo Clin. Proc.* 2012;87:817-824.

[14] Singh, B., Singh, A., Giri, J., et al. Evaluation of digital signature of Charlson comorbidities using automatic electronic note search strategies in critically ill patients. *Crit. Care Med.* 2011;39:160.

[15] American College of Chest Physicians/Society of Critical Care Medicine Consensus Conference: definitions for sepsis and organ failure and guidelines for the use of innovative therapies in sepsis. *Crit. Care Med.* 1992;20:864-874.

[16] Levy, M. M., Fink, M. P., Marshall, J. C., et al. 2001 SCCM/ESICM/ ACCP/ATS/SIS International Sepsis Definitions Conference. *Crit. Care Med.* 2003;31:1250-1256.

[17] Antonelli, M., Levy, M., Andrews, P. J., et al. Hemodynamic monitoring in shock and implications for management. International Consensus Conference, Paris, France, 27-28 April 2006. *Intensive Care Med.* 2007; 33:575-590.

[18] Bernard, G. R., Artigas, A., Brigham, K. L., et al. The American-European Consensus Conference on ARDS. Definitions, mechanisms, relevant outcomes, and clinical trial coordination. *Am. J. Respir. Crit. Care Med.* 1994;149:818-824.

[19] Trey, C., CS. D. The management of fulminant hepatic failure. In: Popper, H., Schaffner, F., eds. *Progress in Liver Diseases,* New York: Grune and Stratton 1970:282–298.

[20] Esteban, A., Anzueto, A., Frutos, F., et al. Characteristics and outcomes in adult patients receiving mechanical ventilation: a 28-day international study. *JAMA* 2002;287:345-355.

[21] Bellomo, R., Ronco, C., Kellum, J. A., et al. Acute renal failure - definition, outcome measures, animal models, fluid therapy and information technology needs: the Second International Consensus Conference of the Acute Dialysis Quality Initiative (ADQI) Group. *Crit. Care* 2004;8:R204-212.

[22] Ranieri, V. M., Thompson, B. T., Barie, P. S., et al. Drotrecogin alfa (activated) in adults with septic shock. *N Eng. J. Med.* 2012;366:2055-2064.

[23] Dhainaut, J. F., Yan, S. B., Joyce, D. E., et al. Treatment effects of drotrecogin alfa (activated) in patients with severe sepsis with or without overt disseminated intravascular coagulation. *J. Thromb. Haemost.* 2004; 2:1924-1933.

[24] Chen, K. T., Lin, H. J., Lee, W. J. Severe disseminated intravascular coagulation caused by congestive heart failure and left ventricular thrombus. *Eur. J. Emerg. Med.* 2007;14:87-89.

[25] Jafri, S. M., Ozawa, T., Mammen, E., et al. Platelet function, thrombin and fibrinolytic activity in patients with heart failure. *European heart journal* 1993;14:205-212.

[26] Cugno, M., Mari, D., Meroni, P. L., et al. Haemostatic and inflammatory biomarkers in advanced chronic heart failure: role of oral anticoagulants and successful heart transplantation. *British journal of haematology* 2004;126:85-92.

[27] Bernard, G. R., Vincent, J. L., Laterre, P. F., et al. Efficacy and safety of recombinant human activated protein C for severe sepsis. *N Engl. J. Med.* 2001;344:699-709.

[28] Vincent, J. L. The rise and fall of drotrecogin alfa (activated). *Lancet Infect. Dis.* 2012.

[29] Kalil, A. C., Larosa, S. P. Effectiveness and safety of drotrecogin alfa (activated) for severe sepsis: a meta-analysis and metaregression. *Lancet Infect. Dis.* 2012.

[30] Abraham, E., Laterre, P. F., Garg, R., et al. Drotrecogin alfa (activated) for adults with severe sepsis and a low risk of death. *The New England journal of medicine* 2005;353:1332-1341.

[31] Balk, R. A. Pathogenesis and management of multiple organ dysfunction or failure in severe sepsis and septic shock. *Crit. Care Clin.* 2000;16: 337-352, vii.

[32] Gando, S., Nanzaki, S., Morimoto, Y., et al. Tissue factor pathway inhibitor response does not correlate with tissue factor-induced disseminated intravascular coagulation and multiple organ dysfunction syndrome in trauma patients. *Crit. Care Med.* 2001;29:262-266.

[33] Ince, C. The microcirculation is the motor of sepsis. *Crit. Care* 2005;9 Suppl. 4:S13-19.

[34] Ruf, W., Riewald, M. Tissue factor-dependent coagulation protease signaling in acute lung injury. *Crit. Care Med.* 2003;31:S231-237.

[35] St. Sauver, J. L., Grossardt, B. R., Leibson, C. L., et al. Generalizability of epidemiological findings and public health decisions: an illustration from the Rochester Epidemiology Project. *Mayo Clin. Proc.* 2012;87: 151-160.

In: Disseminated Intravascular Coagulation (DIC)   ISBN: 978-1-62948-323-8
Editor: Balwinder Singh   © 2014 Nova Science Publishers, Inc.

Chapter VI

Sepsis and Disseminated Intravascular Coagulation

Luis Aurelio Diaz Caballero, MD[*]

Division of Pulmonary and Critical Care Medicine,
Mayo Clinic, Rochester, MN, US

Abstract

Severe sepsis and septic shock remain significant health care problems worldwide and the leading cause of infection-associated mortality among critically ill patients. Recent epidemiological studies estimate the incidence of sepsis to be 3.0 cases per 1,000 population (2.26 cases per 100 hospital discharges) translating to an approximate 750,000 cases and 215,000 deaths (28.6% mortality) annually in the United States alone. Despite numerous advances in early recognition and intervention, the mortality rate for septic shock remains unacceptably high, between 40% and 70%.

The spectrum of sepsis and shock is defined by: (1) A robust systemic inflammatory response to infection, either culture-proven or clinically suspected, (2) The presence or absence of organ dysfunction, and (3) The ability of the host to compensate for such insults. Without an adequate response to fluid and resuscitative efforts, the acute organ dysfunction of severe sepsis may rapidly progress to septic shock. The

---

[*] Email: luisaureliodiaz@gmail.com.

inflammatory response to infection, including endotoxin and exotoxin-mediated cytokine effects upon fibrinolytic and coagulation cascades may result in sepsis-associated coagulopathy. The main mechanisms include up-regulation of procoagulant pathways, the tissue factor (TF) pathway; impaired function of natural anticoagulants, and inhibition of fibrinolysis. Dysregulation may range from subtle hemostatic changes to widespread microvascular thrombosis and disseminated intravascular coagulation (DIC). DIC is an important and independent predictor of progressive organ dysfunction and mortality in patients with sepsis.

Inappropriate initiation of coagulation during sepsis is dependent on expression of TF on circulating monocytes, tissue macrophages and endothelial cells. TF drives thrombin generation, fibrin formation and deposition, and there is evidence that this procoagulant response is followed by an early fibrinolysis due to increased expression of at least two types of plasminogen activators. In sepsis, fibrinolysis is rapidly attenuated by the release of plasminogen activator inhibitor, type 1 (PAI-1).

The resulting effect is a complete inhibition of fibrinolysis causing a net procoagulant state, contributing to microvascular thrombosis. Procoagulant activity is regulated by three natural anticoagulant pathways: Antithrombin (AT), activated protein C (APC), and tissue factor pathway inhibitor (TFPI). Sepsis attenuates the function of all three pathways.

The treatment of sepsis-associated DIC requires: (1) Early recognition and treatment of the underlying infection, including source control as necessary, (2) Early recognition and diagnosis of DIC, (3) Multiple organ supportive therapy and correction of coagulopathies. Experimental and clinical evidence of the anti-inflammatory properties of natural anticoagulants, suggested their potential as a therapeutic strategy to treat severe sepsis. Unfortunately, despite promising results from initial studies, randomized controlled trials utilizing AT, APC and TFPI to reduce sepsis-related mortality have failed to show significant reduction of mortality of patients with sepsis. Moreover, recombinant APC was withdrawn from the market by November 2011 after a randomized trial found no benefit in treated patients. Additional basic and clinical investigations are needed to better identify and evaluate specific treatments of sepsis-associated DIC.

Keywords: Severe sepsis, disseminated intravascular coagulation, intensive care unit, critically ill patient, infection, inflammation, tissue factor, fibrinolysis, natural anticoagulants, antithrombin, activated protein C, tissue factor pathway inhibitor, thrombomodulin

Introduction

Sepsis is defined by the presence of presumed or documented infection associated with systemic manifestations such as fever or hypothermia, tachycardia, tachypnea, leukocytosis, leukopenia, or the presence of immature neutrophils, altered mental status, or hyperlactatemia, among others (Table 1) [1]. Through a series of pathogenic events sepsis may evolve to severe sepsis (acute organ dysfunction secondary to proven or suspected infection) and septic shock (severe sepsis plus hypotension not reversed with fluid resuscitation). The septic response involves a highly complex cross talk between immune, neuroendocrine, and coagulation systems leading to a robust systemic inflammatory response, enhanced coagulation, impaired fibrinolysis, and consumption of coagulation inhibitors [2]. Activation of the inflammatory response leads to dysregulation of the hemostatic system ranging from subclinical activation of coagulation to disseminated intravascular coagulation (DIC). Sepsis-associated coagulopathy can result in inadequate fibrin removal, fibrin deposition in the microvasculature, and widespread microvascular thrombosis, resulting in progressive organ dysfunction, and death. At the same time, the persistent consumption of platelets and coagulation proteins may result in bleeding of varying severity and origin. There is ample evidence that DIC is an important and independent predictor of organ failure and mortality in patients with sepsis [3, 4]. The purpose of this chapter is to review the pathophysiologic bases of sepsis-associated DIC and the therapeutic implications of the cross talk between inflammation and coagulation.

Epidemiology

The incidence of sepsis is currently about 750,000 cases annually in the United States and incidence continues to trend upward. Between 1979 and 2000 the diagnosis of sepsis increased from 82.7 cases per 100,000 to 240.4 cases per 100,000, or an annualized increase of 8.7 percent [5]. The mortality rate associated with severe sepsis or septic shock remains between 30% and 70%. Even single organ dysfunction places patients at a significant risk for dying, with mortality rates increasing approximately 15% to 20% for each additional dysfunctional organ. Mortality rates are highest (ranging from 50% to 80%) for patients with cardiovascular compromise (septic shock) despite aggressive medical care. [5-7].

Table 1. Diagnostic criteria for sepsis in adults

1. Infection: presumed or documented infection associated with some of the following:

2. General variables
>Fever: temperature > 38.3 ° C
>Hypothermia: temperature < 36° C
>Tachycardia: heart rate > 90 per minute
>Tachypnea
>Altered mental status
>Edema or positive fluid balance: > 20 ml/kg over 24 hours
>Hyperglycemia: plasma glucose > 140 mg/dL in the absence of
diabetes

3. Inflammatory variables
>Leukocytosis: WBC count > 12,000 μL^{-1}
>Leukopenia: WBC count < 4,000 μL^{-1}
>Normal WBC count with > 10% immature forms
>Plasma C-reactive protein more than 2 SD above the normal value
>Plasma procalcitonin more than 2 SD above the normal value

4. Hemodynamic variables
>Arterial hypotension: SBP < 90 mm Hg, MAP < 70 mm Hg or an
SBP decrease > 40mmHg

5. Organ dysfunction variables
>Arterial hypoxemia: PaO_2 / FiO_2 < 300
>Acute oliguria: UO < 0.5 mL/kg/hour for at least 2 hours despite fluid
resuscitation
>Creatinine increase > 0.5 mg/dL
>Coagulation abnormalities: INR > 1.5 or aPTT > 60 seconds
>Ileus: Absent bowel sounds
>Thrombocytopenia: platelet count < 100,000 μL^{-1}
>Hyperbilirubinemia: plasma total bilirubin > 4 mg/dL

6. Tissue perfusion variables
>Hyperlactatemia: > 1 mmol/L
>Decreased capillary refill or mottling

[a] PTT=activated partial thromboplastin time; INR=international normalized ratio; MAP=mean arterial pressure; SBP=systolic blood pressure; SD=standard deviation; UO=urine output; WBC=white blood cell. Adapted from Dellinger et al. [1].

Table 2. Diagnostic criteria for overt DIC by the International Society on Thrombosis and Hemostasis

Risk assessment	Patient with underlying disorder compatible with DIC = Yes		
Variables	0 points	1 point	2 points
Platelet count	> 100,000	< 100,000	< 50,000
Elevated fibrin marker	No increase	Moderate increase	Strong increase
Prothrombin time	< 3 seconds	< 6 seconds	> 6 seconds
Fibrinogen level	> 1.0 g/L	< 1.0 g/L	

A score of ≥ 5 is indicative of overt DIC.

DIC frequently complicates sepsis [8]. The International Society of Thrombosis and Hemostasis has proposed a scoring system for overt DIC (Table 2) [9]. Using these criteria, the diagnosis of overt DIC occurs in 25 to 50% of all patients with severe sepsis [3, 4], and is strongly correlated with morbidity and mortality [8]. In patients with sepsis-associated DIC the mortality rate is estimated to be 40%, compared to 27% in patients without DIC [4, 10]. Compared to trauma-associated DIC, patients with sepsis-associated DIC also have a higher mortality [11].

Physiological Hemostatic Response

Hemostasis is a highly complex and regulated process that maintains blood in a fluid state, controls bleeding, and preserves vascular integrity under normal physiologic conditions. Hemostasis is achieved through the interaction of platelet activation, blood clotting, and vascular repair. Two key components contribute to hemostasis.

The first involves interaction between vascular endothelial cells and platelets to culminate in the formation of a platelet plug at the site of injury [12]. The area of endothelial injury provides binding sites for Von Willebrand

Factor through the platelet glycoprotein 1b/IX/V complex and fibrinogen via integrin receptors [13]. The core of the plug is a platelet-ligand-platelet matrix with fibrinogen, fibronectin, and Von Willebrand Factor (vWF) as bridging ligands. The platelet-mediated plug formation is not sufficient for stable hemostasis.

The second component of hemostasis is the coagulation system and the formation of a stable fibrin clot. The initial platelet plug is stabilized by fibrin generated by the coagulation cascade. Fibrin links platelets and provides structural support to the blood clot. Tissue Factor (TF) triggers the coagulation system.

The initiation phase starts as the exposed TF forms a complex with coagulation Factor VIIa (FVIIa). FVIIa is normally circulated in a biologically inactive form in the picomolar range, until complex formation occurs with TF [14]. This TF-VIIa complex catalyzes the conversion of Factor X (FX) to Factor Xa (FXa), which generates small amounts of thrombin. Balancing this process, there is a rapid inhibition of TF-VIIa complex by the TF pathway inhibitor (TFPI).

Conversely, the indirect pathway also activated by TF-VIIa complex is not inhibited by TFPI. This cascade converts Factor IX (FIX) to Factor IXa (FIXa), and along Factor VIIIa (FVIIIa), converts FX to FXa. Although the formation of thrombin by this pathway is small – and insufficient to transform fibrinogen to fibrin – it sparks the initiation of the propagation phase. Thrombin generated during the initiation phase amplifies the coagulation signal by activating Factor XI, Factor VIII, Factor V, Factor XI, and platelets. This feedback sustains coagulation after TF-VIIa complex is inhibited by TFPI. Successful completion of the propagation phase ends in significant thrombin generation and fibrin deposition (Figure 1) [15].

At the same time, there are two processes to control procoagulant activities: The natural anticoagulant system and the fibrinolytic system. Natural anticoagulants, most importantly TFPI and antithrombin (AT), can prevent the formation of, or inactivate, thrombin, respectively. The elimination phase, the fibrinolytic system, is the last step in the coagulation system. Its main function is the conversion of plasminogen to plasmin by the tissue plasminogen activator (tPA), and is regulated by plasma mediators that inactivate formed plasmin (α2-antiplasmin) or block plasmin generation (plasminogen activator inhibitor-1 (PAI-1)).Both systems are important in limiting clot formation and fibrin deposition to areas of vascular injury. Any dysregulation of the hemostatic system due to infection, cancer trauma, or other insult, may lead to DIC.

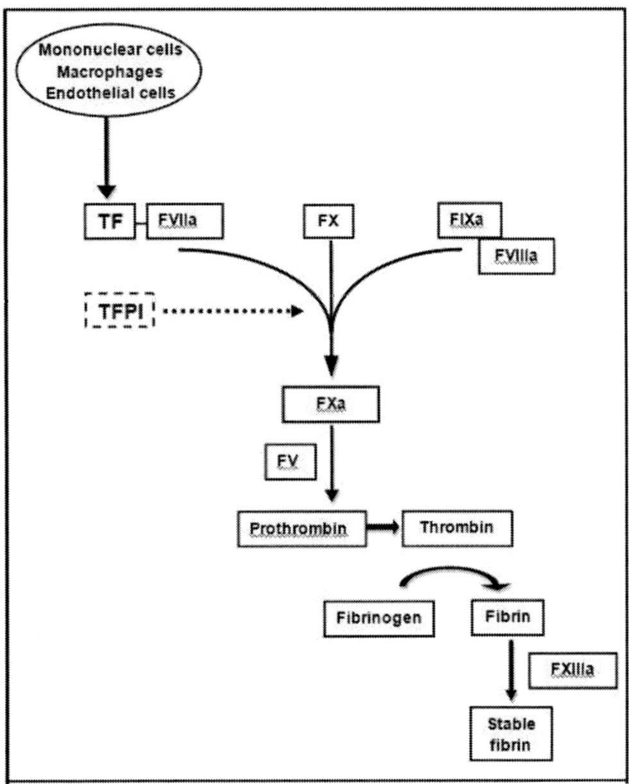

FV: Factor V, FVIIa: Activates Factor VII, FVIIIa: Activated Factor VIII, FX: Factor X, FXa: Activated Factor X, FIXa: Activated Factor IX, FXIIIa: Activated Factor XIII, TF: Tissue Factor, TEPL: Tissue Factor Pathway Inhibitor.

Figure 1. Coagulation Cascade.

Pathogenesis of Sepsis-Associated DIC

The main mechanisms of sepsis-associated coagulopathy are up-regulation of procoagulant pathways, impaired function of natural anticoagulants, and inhibition of fibrinolysis. In severe sepsis, the causative organism triggers a systemic inflammatory response which leads to the generation of proinflammatory cytokines that act in concert with the offending organism and/or associated endotoxins or exotoxins, to elicit the coagulation and fibrinolytic pathways. These processes are principally regulated by interleukin (IL)-1, IL-6, and tumor necrosis factor (TNF)-α [16], that, in turn, stimulate endothelial cells and monocytes to express TF. Initiation of coagulation during sepsis is dependent on expression of TF on circulating monocytes, tissue macrophages and endothelial cells which drive thrombin generation, fibrin formation and deposition [17, 18]. The essential role of TF exposure in the development of DIC was demonstrated in baboon models of severe sepsis [19, 20]. In these studies, the inhibition of TF diminished the inflammatory response, the intensity of DIC and the dysfunction of several organs.

Three natural anticoagulant pathways oppose the activation of coagulation: Antithrombin (AT), activated protein C (APC), and tissue factor pathway inhibitor (TFPI). AT rapidly inactivates thrombin by creating thrombin-antithrombin (TAT) complexes, which are then cleared from circulation. Thrombomodulin (TM) also binds thrombin, inhibiting its procoagulant activity. This thrombin-TM (TTM) complex also activates protein C, inactivating the essential coagulation factors Va and VIIIa, acting and thus acts as an efficient anticoagulant by diminishing thrombin generation. Marked reduction in plasma levels of AT occur during sepsis due to the decreased hepatic synthesis and increased clearance of TAT complexes [21, 22]. There is evidence that the second natural anticoagulant, APC, plays a key role in the pathogenesis of sepsis-associated organ dysfunction and coagulopathy [23, 24]. Activity of the APC system is significantly reduced due to low levels of protein C and S [25, 26] and down-regulation of TM. The third natural anticoagulant, TFPI, inhibits TF-VIIa complex by forming a quaternary complex with FXa. In patients with DIC there is an elevated TF level, suggesting a relative TFPI insufficiency that results in unchallenged thrombin generation [27]. Sepsis attenuates the function of all three of these pathways, resulting in a net procoagulant state.

After the activation of the TF procoagulant pathway there is an early fibrinolysis due to increased expression of at least two types of plasminogen activators: Tissue-type plasminogen activator (t-PA) and urokinase-like plasminogen activator (u-PA) [28]. In sepsis, endotoxins, TNF-α, and IL-1 induce the release of plasminogen activator inhibitor, type 1 (PAI-1) that rapidly attenuates fibrinolysis [29, 30]. PAI-1 can inactivate both plasminogen activators by forming stable complexes with either t-PA or u-PA [29]. Another mechanism for fibrinolysis dysfunction is α-2 antiplasmin which inactivates plasmin by forming plasmin-α-2 antiplasmin complexes [29]. The resulting effect is a complete inhibition of fibrinolysis contributing to microvascular thrombosis. In DIC, the rapid activation of the coagulation cascade results in vigorous consumption of coagulation factors and platelets leading to severe bleeding, or even coexisting thrombosis and bleeding [31].

Inflammation and Coagulation Cross-Talk in DIC

The relation between inflammation and coagulation is bidirectional, and coagulation can also regulate inflammatory activity. There is a significant interaction between coagulation proteases and protease inhibitors with specific cell receptors on monocytes and endothelial cells that may modulate cytokine production or inflammatory processes [32]. TF-VIIa complex, FXa, and thrombin can induce pro-inflammatory activities [33]. Thrombin stimulates IL-1 production from macrophages; FXa, thrombin, and fibrin can elicit the production of IL-6 and IL-8 [33]. AT has important anti-inflammatory properties [34], predominately through the attenuation of thrombin activity. Thrombin activates endothelial cells and platelets which contribute to local inflammation [35].

Activated platelets release inflammatory mediators to stimulate leukocyte activity, all these pro-inflammatory responses are inhibited by AT. There is ample evidence that the APC system, in addition to its role as a coagulation modulator, regulates inflammation [36, 37]. APC has anti-inflammatory effects on monocytes and granulocytes by binding to the endothelial protein C receptor (EPCR), activating protease activated receptor, type 1 (PAR-1), and inhibiting inflammation and apoptosis [38]. In experiments with septic baboons, the blockage of the protein C pathway increased the inflammatory response, and this was attenuated by the administration of APC [39]. In sepsis-associated DIC, there is an insufficient response of anti-inflammatory cytokines (IL-1 receptor antagonist, IL-4, IL-10, IL-13, and soluble TNFα receptors) to overcome the broad inflammatory response in multiple organs [40].

Diagnostic Criteria for DIC

In severe sepsis, activation of inflammatory and coagulation responses lead to hemostatic abnormalities ranging from subtle activation of coagulation to DIC. Patients with sepsis-associated DIC present with multiple organ dysfunction syndrome (MODS), which is the main cause of mortality [41]. A myriad of laboratory abnormalities can be found in sepsis-associated DIC, the most common of which is thrombocytopenia, although prolonged prothrombin time (PT), reduction in fibrinogen, and an increase in fibrin degradation products (FDP) are also frequently observed. Thrombocytopenia correlates with thrombin production and is an indicator of the severity of DIC [13, 42]; nonetheless, the thrombocytopenia of sepsis-induced DIC must be distinguished from other causes, including thrombotic thrombocytopenic purpura, liver cirrhosis, medications, radiotherapy, bone marrow suppression, or anti-platelets antibodies, among others.

In DIC, thrombocytopenia is a result of platelet activation and consumption, suppression of bone marrow platelet production, and enhanced clearance by the reticuloendothelial system [13]. Activated partial thromboplastin time and PT are prolonged in almost 50% of patients due to consumption of coagulant factors, impaired hepatic production, or vitamin K deficiency. But, PT can be prolonged and fibrinogen levels can be reduced in patients with hepatic dysfunction. Alternatively, fibrinogen is an acute phase reactant, and in patients with a strong inflammatory response to infection, fibrinogen level and the platelet levels may be increased, rather than decreased. Global coagulation tests can point toward consumptive coagulopathy, but may be misleading when alternative underlying etiologies are present. Therefore, such studies are not specific for a diagnosis of DIC.

The Scientific Subcommittee on DIC of the International Society on Thrombosis and Haemostasis (ISTH) defined the criteria for overt DIC in 2001 (Table 2) [9]. These criteria were validated in a prospective study and the reported per patient sensitivity was 93% with a specificity of 98% [43]. The prothrombin time and the platelet count are valuable in predicting severity and risk of mortality [44, 45].

Therapeutic Strategies

The keystone of the treatment of sepsis-associated DIC is based upon: (1) Early treatment of the underlying infection, (2) Early diagnosis of DIC, (3) Multiple organ supportive therapy including intervention for coagulation abnormalities.

While the most important interventions for sepsis-associated DIC include the immediate and appropriate antibiotic therapy and source control of the underlying infection while providing appropriate supportive care for multiple organ dysfunctions, a role for adjunctive therapies to manage coagulopathy has been proposed.

Heparin, Platelets, and Coagulation Factors

The anticoagulants unfractionated heparin (UFH), low molecular-weight heparin (LMWH), and dapanaroid sodium modulate the hemostatic abnormalities binding to the enzyme inhibitor antithrombin (AT) causing a conformational change that result in its activation. Although theoretically useful and widely debated, no randomized, controlled clinical trials of the administration of anticoagulants in sepsis-associated DIC have demonstrated a beneficial effect on clinically important outcomes [46]. Additionally, the safety of therapeutic doses of heparins, in patients who have a higher risk of bleeding, remains controversial. In patients with overt thromboembolism, deep vein thrombosis, arterial thrombosis, acral ischemia, or purpura fulminans therapeutic doses of heparins are indicated [42]. Moreover, guidelines recommend the use of prophylactic doses of heparins in DIC [42]. Significant thrombocytopenia and low levels of coagulation factors may increase the risk of bleeding, but substitution therapy is indicated only if there is active bleeding, because the treatment of the underlying cause will correct the hemostatic abnormalities [42, 47]. In patients with specific deficiencies such as fibrinogen, cryoprecipitate is the recommended therapy with a target goal of 1 gram/liter [42]. With regards to Factor VIIa, the evidence to recommend its use is lacking. There are not randomized, controlled trials demonstrating its efficacy [48].

New Strategies: Natural Anticoagulants Therapy

In view of recent advances in our understanding of the pathogenic mechanisms of sepsis-associated DIC, interest has changed from procoagulant replacement to the anticoagulant therapy. As a result, restoration of natural anticoagulant pathways, fibrinolysis, and thereby modulation of the inflammatory response has been an appealing target for new therapeutic strategies. Randomized controlled trials on the efficacy of AT, APC, and TFPI to reduce sepsis-related mortality have been completed [10, 49, 50].

Antithrombin Concentrate in Sepsis-associated DIC

AT is the main inhibitor of thrombin and FXa. Levels of AT are rapidly decreased in early severe sepsis due to formation of complexes between AT and multiple activated clotting factors [51]. In studies of sepsis patients [21, 51, 52], rapid depletion of AT is highly predictive of a fatal outcome. AT replacement consistently improves the outcomes of sepsis in a variety of animal models [53, 54], and this is the therapeutic rationale for the use of AT in severe sepsis and septic shock patients. Initial trials of AT therapy in sepsis revealed promising results [55-59]. In a French, randomized, double-blind placebo-controlled trial of 35 patients with documented septic shock and DIC [55], the treatment group received AT (90 to 120 IU/kg in loading dose, then 90 to 120 IU/kg/d during 4 days). The treatment group had a significant reduction in the duration of DIC, while the observed 44% reduction in ICU mortality did not reach statistical significance. In a randomized, prospective study [56] to determine whether long-term AT supplementation had beneficial effects on organ function, 40 consecutive surgical patients with severe sepsis were randomized to either placebo or AT, and the treatment group received a 14-day continuous infusion to obtain plasma AT activities > 120%. Findings suggested that supplementation with AT may improve lung function, attenuate DIC, and prevent the development of liver and kidney dysfunction in patients with severe sepsis, but no difference in mortality was observed. A double-blind, randomized, multicenter study [58], including 120 patients admitted to the ICU with low levels of AT (including 56 patients in septic shock) were randomized to receive AT (total dose 24000 units) or placebo treatment for 5 days. Although no overall survival benefit was found, subgroup analysis of replacement therapy with AT in patients with septic shock appeared to reduce mortality [58]. In a review of the literature from 1966 to 1998, Levi et al. [60] assessed the effect of AT on mortality in patients with sepsis and DIC. They performed a meta-analysis of randomized controlled trials, and observed a statistically significant reduction in mortality (from 47% to 32%, odds ratio, 0.59; 95% confidence interval, 0.39-0.87).

Based on the promising results of experimental and small clinical trials, a large-scale, double-blind, multicenter, randomized controlled trial (High-dose antithrombin in severe sepsis – the KYBERSEPT trial) [49] addressed the effect on survival of high-dose antithrombin (administered within 6 hours of onset) in patients with severe sepsis and septic shock. The study included 2,314 adult patients, randomized to receive either intravenous antithrombin (30,000 IU in total over 4 days) or a placebo (1% human albumin). The protocol allowed low doses of heparin for prophylaxis (≤10.000 IU/d) and heparin flushes for catheter patency.

The mortality rate for the group treated with AT concentrate was 38.9 % compared to a mortality rate of 38.7 % for the placebo group (p=0.94).

Moreover, the treatment group had more significant bleeding complications compared to placebo (23.8% versus 13.5%). Unexpectedly, subgroup analysis showed a trend toward a survival benefit at 28 days in patients who did not receive concomitant heparin and who met ISTH criteria for overt DIC (Relative mortality risk reduction ~15%) and this trend became statistically significant at 90 days [49]. A proposed explanation for this finding may be that heparin antagonizes the microcirculatory and anti-inflammatory effects of AT [37], as evidenced in animal models of sepsis [61]. The potential benefit of AT treatment on patients with severe sepsis and DIC remains unclear and should be investigated in prospective trials.

Recombinant Tissue Factor Pathway Inhibitor in Sepsis-Associated DIC

TFPI is an endogenous inhibitor of the TF pathway of blood coagulation. TFPI forms an inhibitory complex with TF, FVIIa, and FXa, blocking the conversion of prothrombin from thrombin. Theoretically, TF inhibitors ought to be efficacious in sepsis-associated DIC given the central role of TF/FVIIa pathway in the activation of coagulation. In terms of preventing thrombin generation, TFPI may inhibit the coagulation cascade at a proximal point compared with other antithrombotic agents. Recombinant protein TFPI (rTFPI) differs from the native protein by a single additional alanine residue at the amino terminus. In animal models of severe sepsis, including lethal intravenous Escherichia coli infusion in baboons [62, 63], the administration of rTFPI attenuated the coagulopathic response, decreased organ dysfunction, circulating levels of cytokines and improved survival. These studies showed that administration of rTFPI, even several hours after infectious challenge, could improve outcome. In a phase two, prospective, randomized, single-blind, placebo-controlled, dose escalation, multicenter trial [64], of 210 patients with severe sepsis, the continuous intravenous infusion of placebo or rTFPI at 0.025 or 0.05 mg/kg/hr for 4 days (96 hrs) reduced the coagulant and the inflammatory responses.

The study showed a trend toward reduction in 28-day all-cause mortality in the treatment arm, and demonstrated that rTFPI doses of 0.025 and 0.05 mg/kg/hr could be safely administered to severe sepsis patients.

Based on the beneficial results in human phase one and phase two trials [62, 64, 65], a phase three randomized, double-blind, placebo-controlled, multicenter clinical trial (OPTIMIST trial) [50] was performed. The aims of the study were to assess the efficacy of rTFPI in patients with severe sepsis and high international normalized ratio (INR) ($\geq$1.2) and to evaluate rTFPI safety in severe sepsis, including patients with low INR. 1,754 patients with an INR $\geq$1.2 and 201 patients with an INR <1.2 were assigned to intravenous infusion of either rTFPI (0.025 mg/kg per hour for 96 hours, n = 880) or placebo. rTFPI significantly attenuated the coagulopathic response in both groups, but the overall mortality at 28 days in the treated group (n = 880) versus the placebo group (n = 874) for high INR was 34.2% versus 33.9%, respectively (p =0.88).

Furthermore, there was a significant increase in risk of bleeding in the treated group, irrespective of baseline INR [50]. In the rTFPI trials there was no difference in the mortality rate in the treatment groups with or without heparin, in contrast to the KYBERSEPT trial [49] where heparin may have interfered with the beneficial effects of AT concentrate; administration of heparin does not appear to explain this trial outcome [50]. A subgroup analysis of the OPTIMIST trial [50] showed a trend toward improved survival in patients with severe community acquired pneumonia treated with rTFPI (mortality rate 27.9% versus 32.7%; p = 0.25).

The benefit was larger when only severe community acquired pneumonia patients with a microbiologically identified infection were included in the analysis (mortality rate with rTFPI 27.1%, versus 35.7% with placebo; p = 0.09). Given these findings, the multicenter, randomized, placebo-controlled, double-blind, three-arm study CAPTIVATE trial was conducted [66]. Its goal was to assess the efficacy of adjunctive rTFPI in patients with severe community acquired pneumonia. 2,138 patients were included in the trial, 946, 238, and 918 received rTFPI 0.025 mg/kg/h, rTFPI 0.075 mg/kg/h, and placebo, respectively.

The use of heparin was not allowed during the infusion of rTFPI. The trial arm receiving rTFPI infusion at 0.075 mg/kg/hour was stopped early for futility. CAPTIVATE demonstrated no mortality benefit in patients with severe community acquired pneumonia despite evidence of pharmacodynamic effect, although it should be noted that the proportion of patients with sepsis-associated DIC was only 4.8% [66]. Nonetheless, the conclusion from this recent and well-conducted study is that the administration of rTFPI provides no significant benefit to patients with severe community acquired pneumonia or sepsis.

Recombinant Human Activated Protein C in Sepsis-Associated DIC

Protein C is the zymogen of the protease activated protein C (APC). The complex thrombin-thrombomodulin (TTM) activates protein C. By inactivating coagulation factors Va and VIIIa, diminishing thrombin generation, APC is an efficient anticoagulant. Moreover, APC increases fibrinolytic activity and modulates the inflammatory response [51]. Based on the concept that depletion of the protein C system may be critical to the pathophysiology of sepsis-associated DIC, pharmacologic substitution of APC had been investigated as a promising therapy. In early animal models of sepsis [39] and in human phase two trial, recombinant human APC (rhAPC) decreased organ dysfunction, coagulopathy and death [70]. In several randomized controlled trials rhAPC demonstrated a reduction in 28-day mortality [50, 67-69].

The landmark phase three PROWESS trial [10] – a randomized, double-blind, placebo-controlled, multicenter study – included 1,690 patients with severe sepsis and found a significant reduction in all-cause mortality in those patients receiving rhAPC (30.8 % placebo versus 24.7 % rhAPC, absolute risk reduction of death 6.1 %, p=0.005). The incidence of serious bleeding events was higher in the rhAPC group compared to placebo group but this difference was not statistically significant (3.5 % versus 2.0 %, p=0.06). This was the first clinical trial demonstrating a significant reduction of mortality in patients with severe sepsis. As a result, the use of rhAPC in patients with severe sepsis and multiorgan dysfunction was advocated in the guidelines for the treatment of sepsis [71]. Several secondary analyses followed the publication of the PROWESS trial, and demonstrated that patients with the most severe multiorgan dysfunction derived the greatest benefit [72].

However, the role of rhAPC in sepsis remained controversial following the publication of several negative studies [68, 69, 73, 74]. A recent Cochrane Systematic Review [73], including 5 randomized controlled trials and 5,101 adult and pediatric patients with severe sepsis, showed that the administration of rhAPC did not reduce the risk of death at 28 days and increased the risk of bleeding (p=0.001). A prior meta-analysis concluded that, even in severely ill patients, the basis for treatment with rhAPC was not strong or even insufficient [74]; Clinical trials in specific populations of patients with severe sepsis did not show benefit in the 28-day mortality (ADDRESS [68], and XPRESS trials [69]). In view of the conflicting reports of the efficacy of rhAPC, its exact role in the treatment of sepsis was debated for more than a decade, and unresolved criticisms including the possibility of bleeding complications culminated in the manufacturer-sponsored randomized, multinational, placebo-controlled, double-blind study to evaluate the effectiveness of rhAPC in patients with septic shock (PROWESS-SHOCK trial) [75]. This study included 1,697 patients with septic shock who were receiving fluids and vasopressors above a threshold dose for 4 hours to receive either rhAPC (at a dose of 24 µg per kilogram of body weight per hour) or placebo for 96 hours. At 28 days the mortality rate did not differ significantly between the two groups (26.4 % in the rhAPC group versus 24.2 % in the placebo group (relative risk in the rhAPC group, 1.09; 95% confidence interval 0.92 to 1.28; p=0.31). Significant bleeding complications occurred in 10 patients in the rhAPC group versus 8 in the placebo group (p=0.81). Shortly after this trial the production of rhAPC was discontinued and by November 2011 was withdrawn from the market. An editorial to the study's publication suggested that this well conducted study should end any further pursuit of a niche for rhAPC in the treatment of sepsis [76], however limited studies in certain subpopulation continue to be considered today.

Recombinant Human Soluble Thrombomodulin in Sepsis-Associated DIC

TM is an endothelial anticoagulant factor. TM binds to thrombin and this complex activates protein C, which plays an important role in the inhibition of the anticoagulant and anti-inflammatory response [77]. TM suppresses the production of inflammatory cytokines, such as TNFα and IL-1β, via activated protein C [77]. In sepsis, the expression of TM is downregulated [25, 26, 78] and its replacement is considered a therapeutic strategy. Recombinant human soluble TM (rhTM) has been evaluated in animal models of severe sepsis [79, 80]. These studies showed a marked reduction of liver dysfunction and mortality even with delayed treatment of rhTM, concluding that the administration of rhTM may be a beneficial treatment for septic patients [80]. In a phase three randomized, double-blind clinical trial including 232 patients with DIC complicated hematological malignancies (n=131) or infection (n=101) [81], the administration of rhTM had a significantly better outcome on DIC recovery rate (66.1% in the rhTM group versus 49.9% in the heparin group), but the mortality rate at 28 days was similar (28% in the rhTM group versus 34.6% in the low-dose heparin group). A phase two randomized, double-blind, placebo controlled, multicenter trial, involved 750 septic patients with documented or high risk of overt DIC, evaluated the safety and efficacy of rhTM or placebo for 6 days [82]. The 28-day mortality rate was 17.8% in the treatment group versus 21.6% in the placebo group (p=0.273), which met the pre-specified target of p<0.3 for evidence suggestive of efficacy. A subgroup analyses suggested that patients with sepsis, organ dysfunction, and coagulopathy (INR > 1.4 and low platelet count) are most likely to benefit from treatment with rhTM. Mortality rate was lower in the rhTM group but the difference was not statistical significant [82]. Based on these results, a phase three randomized, double-blind, placebo-controlled, trial is currently underway in the United States to evaluate the safety and efficacy of rhTM in patients with severe sepsis and coagulopathy [83]. The results from this study will hopefully better define the safety and effectiveness of rhTM in the treatment of sepsis-associated DIC.

Conclusion

Significant progress has been made in our understanding of the pathogenic mechanisms underlying sepsis-associated DIC. Laboratory research has revealed the complex mechanisms of physiologic hemostasis and helped develop new therapeutic strategies for the management of patients with severe sepsis and DIC. A multitude of experimental and clinical studies have demonstrated that severe sepsis activates coagulation via TF-Factor VII pathway. Importantly, research has elucidated those constituents of the coagulation system that may have key modulatory roles in the inflammatory response, while emphasizing the extensive cross-talk between the inflammatory and coagulation systems. Experimental studies in animal models of severe sepsis conducted over the last decades had focused on replacement of natural anticoagulants known to be deficient in sepsis. Together with early-phase clinical trials, these findings suggested that the coagulation inhibitors intended to curtail the hematologic and thrombotic complications of DIC might constitute effective therapies for human sepsis. Disappointingly, all randomized clinical trials [49, 50, 66, 75] to date evaluating these natural anticoagulants in patients with sepsis, severe sepsis, and septic shock, have failed to demonstrate a beneficial effect on mortality. The role for these substances remain incompletely understood and the clinical community continues to debate the findings and implications of these studies.

Areas of ongoing controversy include: The limitations of animal models in the exploration of pathogenic mechanisms of human sepsis [84]; The interactions of natural anticoagulants with prophylactic or low-dose heparin [49]; Trial designs that do not take into consideration that activation of coagulation and fibrin formation are a potent innate antibacterial mechanism [85]; The fixed, high dose administration of anticoagulants in most trials irrespective of patient characteristics, time period of sepsis, or degree of coagulation activation [86, 87]. Consequently, alternative anticoagulant therapy for sepsis-associated DIC supported by high-quality evidence does not exist at this time. Since sepsis-associated DIC is multicausal, it is postulated that simultaneous modulation of inflammatory and pro-coagulant response would be more successful. Is there still a place for natural anticoagulants in the treatment of sepsis-associated DIC? The answer to this question requires further study to better determine a potential benefit. Ongoing trials with rhTM and AT hopefully will shed light on this question.

References

[1] Dellinger RP, Levy MM, Rhodes A, Annane D, Gerlach H, Opal SM, Sevransky JE, Sprung CL, Douglas IS, Jaeschke R, Osborn TM, Nunnally ME, Townsend SR, Reinhart K, Kleinpell RM, Angus DC, Deutschman CS, Machado FR, Rubenfeld GD, Webb SA, Beale RJ, Vincent JL, Moreno R. Surviving sepsis campaign: international guidelines for management of severe sepsis and septic shock: 2012. *Crit. Care Med.*, 41(2): 580-637, 2013.

[2] Hotchkiss RS, Karl IE. The pathophysiology and treatment of sepsis. *N. Engl. J. Med.*, 348(2): 138-50, 2003.

[3] Dempfle CE, Wurst M, Smolinski M, Lorenz S, Osika A, Olenik D, Fiedler F, Borggrefe M. Use of soluble fibrin antigen instead of D-dimer as fibrin-related marker may enhance the prognostic power of the ISTH overt DIC score. *Thromb. Haemost.*, 91(4): 812-8, 2004.

[4] Dhainaut JF, Yan SB, Joyce DE, Pettila V, Basson B, Brandt JT, Sundin DP, Levi M. Treatment effects of drotrecogin alfa (activated) in patients with severe sepsis with or without overt disseminated intravascular coagulation. *J. Thromb. Haemost.*, 2(11): 1924-33, 2004.

[5] Angus DC, Linde-Zwirble WT, Lidicker J, Clermont G, Carcillo J, Pinsky MR. Epidemiology of severe sepsis in the United States: analysis

of incidence, outcome, and associated costs of care. *Crit. Care Med.,* 29(7): 1303-10, 2001.

[6] Sasse KC, Nauenberg E, Long A, Anton B, Tucker HJ, Hu TW. Long-term survival after intensive care unit admission with sepsis. *Crit. Care Med.,* 23(6): 1040-7, 1995.

[7] Annane D, Aegerter P, Jars-Guincestre MC, Guidet B. Current epidemiology of septic shock: the CUB-Rea Network. *Am. J. Respir. Crit. Care Med.,* 168(2): 165-72, 2003.

[8] Ogura H, Gando S, Iba T, Eguchi Y, Ohtomo Y, Okamoto K, Koseki K, Mayumi T, Murata A, Ikeda T, Ishikura H, Ueyama M, Kushimoto S, Saitoh D, Endo S, Shimazaki S. SIRS-associated coagulopathy and organ dysfunction in critically ill patients with thrombocytopenia. *Shock,* 28(4): 411-7, 2007.

[9] Taylor FB, Jr., Toh CH, Hoots WK, Wada H, Levi M. Towards definition, clinical and laboratory criteria, and a scoring system for disseminated intravascular coagulation. *Thromb. Haemost,* 86(5): 1327-30, 2001.

[10] Bernard GR, Vincent JL, Laterre PF, LaRosa SP, Dhainaut JF, Lopez-Rodriguez A, Steingrub JS, Garber GE, Helterbrand JD, Ely EW, Fisher CJ, Jr. Efficacy and safety of recombinant human activated protein C for severe sepsis. *N. Engl. J. Med.,* 344(10): 699-709, 2001.

[11] Kushimoto S, Gando S, Saitoh D, Ogura H, Mayumi T, Koseki K, Ikeda T, Ishikura H, Iba T, Ueyama M, Eguchi Y, Otomo Y, Okamoto K, Endo S, Shimazaki S. Clinical course and outcome of disseminated intravascular coagulation diagnosed by Japanese Association for Acute Medicine criteria. Comparison between sepsis and trauma. *Thromb. Haemost.,* 100(6): 1099-105, 2008.

[12] Watson SP. Collagen receptor signaling in platelets and megakaryocytes. *Thromb. Haemost.,* 82(2): 365-76, 1999.

[13] Levi M. Platelets in sepsis. *Hematology,* 10 Suppl 1(129-31, 2005.

[14] Davizon P, Munday AD, Lopez JA. Tissue factor, lipid rafts, and microparticles. *Semin. Thromb. Hemost.,* 36(8): 857-64.

[15] Brummel-Ziedins K, Vossen CY, Rosendaal FR, Umezaki K, Mann KG. The plasma hemostatic proteome: thrombin generation in healthy individuals. *J. Thromb. Haemost.,* 3(7): 1472-81, 2005.

[16] van der Poll T, Buller HR, ten Cate H, Wortel CH, Bauer KA, van Deventer SJ, Hack CE, Sauerwein HP, Rosenberg RD, ten Cate JW. Activation of coagulation after administration of tumor necrosis factor to normal subjects. *N. Engl. J. Med.,* 322(23): 1622-7, 1990.

[17] Franco RF, de Jonge E, Dekkers PE, Timmerman JJ, Spek CA, van Deventer SJ, van Deursen P, van Kerkhoff L, van Gemen B, ten Cate H, van der Poll T, Reitsma PH. The in vivo kinetics of tissue factor messenger RNA expression during human endotoxemia: relationship with activation of coagulation. *Blood,* 96(2): 554-9, 2000.

[18] Aird WC. Vascular bed-specific hemostasis: role of endothelium in sepsis pathogenesis. *Crit. Care Med.,* 29(7 Suppl): S28-34; discussion S34-5, 2001.

[19] Taylor FB, Jr., Chang A, Ruf W, Morrissey JH, Hinshaw L, Catlett R, Blick K, Edgington TS. Lethal E. coli septic shock is prevented by blocking tissue factor with monoclonal antibody. *Circ. Shock,* 33(3): 127-34, 1991.

[20] Silasi-Mansat R, Zhu H, Popescu NI, Peer G, Sfyroera G, Magotti P, Ivanciu L, Lupu C, Mollnes TE, Taylor FB, Kinasewitz G, Lambris JD, Lupu F. Complement inhibition decreases the procoagulant response and confers organ protection in a baboon model of Escherichia coli sepsis. *Blood,* 116(6): 1002-10.

[21] Mesters RM, Mannucci PM, Coppola R, Keller T, Ostermann H, Kienast J. Factor VIIa and antithrombin III activity during severe sepsis and septic shock in neutropenic patients. *Blood,* 88(3): 881-6, 1996.

[22] Niessen RW, Lamping RJ, Jansen PM, Prins MH, Peters M, Taylor FB, Jr., de Vijlder JJ, ten Cate JW, Hack CE, Sturk A. Antithrombin acts as a negative acute phase protein as established with studies on HepG2 cells and in baboons. *Thromb. Haemost.,* 78(3): 1088-92, 1997.

[23] Levi M, van der Poll T. Recombinant human activated protein C: current insights into its mechanism of action. Crit Care 11 Suppl 5(S3, 2007.

[24] Esmon CT. Role of coagulation inhibitors in inflammation. *Thromb. Haemost.,* 86(1): 51-6, 2001.

[25] Vary TC, Kimball SR. Regulation of hepatic protein synthesis in chronic inflammation and sepsis. *Am. J. Physiol.,* 262(2 Pt 1): C445-52, 1992.

[26] Faust SN, Levin M, Harrison OB, Goldin RD, Lockhart MS, Kondaveeti S, Laszik Z, Esmon CT, Heyderman RS. Dysfunction of endothelial protein C activation in severe meningococcal sepsis. *N. Engl. J. Med.,* 345(6): 408-16, 2001.

[27] Asakura H, Ontachi Y, Mizutani T, Kato M, Saito M, Morishita E, Yamazaki M, Suga Y, Takami A, Miyamoto K, Nakao S. Elevated levels of free tissue factor pathway inhibitor antigen in cases of disseminated intravascular coagulation caused by various underlying diseases. *Blood Coagul. Fibrinolysis,* 12(1): 1-8, 2001.

[28] Collen D. The plasminogen (fibrinolytic) system. *Thromb. Haemost.,* 82(2): 259-70, 1999.

[29] Hack CE. Fibrinolysis in disseminated intravascular coagulation. *Semin. Thromb. Hemost.,* 27(6): 633-8, 2001.

[30] Biemond BJ, Levi M, Ten Cate H, Van der Poll T, Buller HR, Hack CE, Ten Cate JW. Plasminogen activator and plasminogen activator inhibitor I release during experimental endotoxaemia in chimpanzees: effect of interventions in the cytokine and coagulation cascades. *Clin. Sci.,* (Lond) 88(5): 587-94, 1995.

[31] Levi M. Current understanding of disseminated intravascular coagulation. *Br. J. Haematol.,* 124(5): 567-76, 2004.

[32] Coughlin SR. Thrombin signalling and protease-activated receptors. *Nature,* 407(6801): 258-64, 2000.

[33] van der Poll T, de Jonge E, Levi M. Regulatory role of cytokines in disseminated intravascular coagulation. *Semin. Thromb. Hemost.,* 27(6): 639-51, 2001.

[34] Roemisch J, Gray E, Hoffmann JN, Wiedermann CJ. Antithrombin: a new look at the actions of a serine protease inhibitor. *Blood Coagul. Fibrinolysis,* 13(8): 657-70, 2002.

[35] Opal SM. Interactions between coagulation and inflammation. *Scand. J. Infect. Dis.,* 35(9): 545-54, 2003.

[36] Harada N, Okajima K, Kushimoto S, Isobe H, Tanaka K. Antithrombin reduces ischemia/reperfusion injury of rat liver by increasing the hepatic level of prostacyclin. *Blood,* 93(1): 157-64, 1999.

[37] Horie S, Ishii H, Kazama M. Heparin-like glycosaminoglycan is a receptor for antithrombin III-dependent but not for thrombin-dependent prostacyclin production in human endothelial cells. *Thromb. Res.,* 59(6): 895-904, 1990.

[38] Rezaie AR. Regulation of the protein C anticoagulant and antiinflammatory pathways. *Curr. Med. Chem.,* 17(19): 2059-69,

[39] Taylor FB, Jr., Chang A, Esmon CT, D'Angelo A, Vigano-D'Angelo S, Blick KE. Protein C prevents the coagulopathic and lethal effects of Escherichia coli infusion in the baboon. *J. Clin. Invest.,* 79(3): 918-25, 1987.

[40] Cavaillon JM, Annane D. Compartmentalization of the inflammatory response in sepsis and SIRS. *J. Endotoxin. Res.,* 12(3): 151-70, 2006.

[41] Semeraro N, Ammollo CT, Semeraro F, Colucci M. Sepsis, thrombosis and organ dysfunction. *Thromb. Res.,* 129(3): 290-5.

[42] Levi M, Toh CH, Thachil J, Watson HG. Guidelines for the diagnosis and management of disseminated intravascular coagulation. British Committee for Standards in Haematology. *Br. J. Haematol.,* 145(1): 24-33, 2009.

[43] Bakhtiari K, Meijers JC, de Jonge E, Levi M. Prospective validation of the International Society of Thrombosis and Haemostasis scoring system for disseminated intravascular coagulation. *Crit. Care Med.,* 32(12): 2416-21, 2004.

[44] Toh CH, Hoots WK. The scoring system of the Scientific and Standardisation Committee on Disseminated Intravascular Coagulation of the International Society on Thrombosis and Haemostasis: a 5-year overview. *J. Thromb. Haemost.,* 5(3): 604-6, 2007.

[45] Voves C, Wuillemin WA, Zeerleder S. International Society on Thrombosis and Haemostasis score for overt disseminated intravascular coagulation predicts organ dysfunction and fatality in sepsis patients. *Blood Coagul. Fibrinolysis,* 17(6): 445-51, 2006.

[46] Feinstein DI. Diagnosis and management of disseminated intravascular coagulation: the role of heparin therapy. *Blood,* 60(2): 284-7, 1982.

[47] Levi M. Disseminated intravascular coagulation. *Crit. Care Med.,* 35(9): 2191-5, 2007.

[48] Franchini M, Manzato F, Salvagno GL, Lippi G. Potential role of recombinant activated factor VII for the treatment of severe bleeding associated with disseminated intravascular coagulation: a systematic review. *Blood Coagul. Fibrinolysis,* 18(7): 589-93, 2007.

[49] Warren BL, Eid A, Singer P, Pillay SS, Carl P, Novak I, Chalupa P, Atherstone A, Penzes I, Kubler A, Knaub S, Keinecke HO, Heinrichs H, Schindel F, Juers M, Bone RC, Opal SM. Caring for the critically ill patient. High-dose antithrombin III in severe sepsis: a randomized controlled trial. *JAMA,* 286(15): 1869-78, 2001.

[50] Abraham E, Reinhart K, Opal S, Demeyer I, Doig C, Rodriguez AL, Beale R, Svoboda P, Laterre PF, Simon S, Light B, Spapen H, Stone J, Seibert A, Peckelsen C, De Deyne C, Postier R, Pettila V, Artigas A, Percell SR, Shu V, Zwingelstein C, Tobias J, Poole L, Stolzenbach JC, Creasey AA. Efficacy and safety of tifacogin (recombinant tissue factor pathway inhibitor) in severe sepsis: a randomized controlled trial. *JAMA,* 290(2): 238-47, 2003.

[51] Vervloet MG, Thijs LG, Hack CE. Derangements of coagulation and fibrinolysis in critically ill patients with sepsis and septic shock. *Semin. Thromb. Hemost.,* 24(1): 33-44, 1998.

[52] Fourrier F, Chopin C, Goudemand J, Hendrycx S, Caron C, Rime A, Marey A, Lestavel P. Septic shock, multiple organ failure, and disseminated intravascular coagulation. Compared patterns of antithrombin III, protein C, and protein S deficiencies. *Chest,* 101(3): 816-23, 1992.

[53] Dickneite G. Antithrombin III in animal models of sepsis and organ failure. *Semin. Thromb. Hemost.,* 24(1): 61-9, 1998.

[54] Mammen EF. Antithrombin: its physiological importance and role in DIC. *Semin. Thromb. Hemost.,* 24(1): 19-25, 1998.

[55] Fourrier F, Chopin C, Huart JJ, Runge I, Caron C, Goudemand J. Double-blind, placebo-controlled trial of antithrombin III concentrates in septic shock with disseminated intravascular coagulation. *Chest,* 104(3): 882-8, 1993.

[56] Inthorn D, Hoffmann JN, Hartl WH, Muhlbayer D, Jochum M. Antithrombin III supplementation in severe sepsis: beneficial effects on organ dysfunction. *Shock,* 8(5): 328-34, 1997.

[57] Eisele B, Lamy M, Thijs LG, Keinecke HO, Schuster HP, Matthias FR, Fourrier F, Heinrichs H, Delvos U. Antithrombin III in patients with severe sepsis. A randomized, placebo-controlled, double-blind multicenter trial plus a meta-analysis on all randomized, placebo-controlled, double-blind trials with antithrombin III in severe sepsis. *Intensive Care Med.,* 24(7): 663-72, 1998.

[58] Baudo F, Caimi TM, de Cataldo F, Ravizza A, Arlati S, Casella G, Carugo D, Palareti G, Legnani C, Ridolfi L, Rossi R, D'Angelo A, Crippa L, Giudici D, Gallioli G, Wolfler A, Calori G. Antithrombin III (ATIII) replacement therapy in patients with sepsis and/or postsurgical complications: a controlled double-blind, randomized, multicenter study. *Intensive Care Med.,* 24(4): 336-42, 1998.

[59] Inthorn D, Hoffmann JN, Hartl WH, Muhlbayer D, Jochum M. Effect of antithrombin III supplementation on inflammatory response in patients with severe sepsis. *Shock,* 10(2): 90-6, 1998.

[60] Levi M, de Jonge E, van der Poll T, ten Cate H. Disseminated intravascular coagulation. Thromb Haemost 82(2): 695-705, 1999.

[61] Hoffmann JN, Vollmar B, Laschke MW, Inthorn D, Kaneider NC, Dunzendorfer S, Wiedermann CJ, Romisch J, Schildberg FW, Menger MD. Adverse effect of heparin on antithrombin action during endotoxemia: microhemodynamic and cellular mechanisms. *Thromb. Haemost.,* 88(2): 242-52, 2002.

[62] Creasey AA, Chang AC, Feigen L, Wun TC, Taylor FB, Jr., Hinshaw LB. Tissue factor pathway inhibitor reduces mortality from Escherichia coli septic shock. *J. Clin. Invest.*, 91(6): 2850-60, 1993.

[63] Carr C, Bild GS, Chang AC, Peer GT, Palmier MO, Frazier RB, Gustafson ME, Wun TC, Creasey AA, Hinshaw LB, et al. Recombinant E. coli-derived tissue factor pathway inhibitor reduces coagulopathic and lethal effects in the baboon gram-negative model of septic shock. *Circ. Shock,* 44(3): 126-37, 1994.

[64] Abraham E, Reinhart K, Svoboda P, Seibert A, Olthoff D, Dal Nogare A, Postier R, Hempelmann G, Butler T, Martin E, Zwingelstein C, Percell S, Shu V, Leighton A, Creasey AA. Assessment of the safety of recombinant tissue factor pathway inhibitor in patients with severe sepsis: a multicenter, randomized, placebo-controlled, single-blind, dose escalation study. *Crit. Care Med.,* 29(11): 2081-9, 2001.

[65] Abraham E. Tissue factor inhibition and clinical trial results of tissue factor pathway inhibitor in sepsis. *Crit. Care Med.,* 28(9 Suppl): S31-3, 2000.

[66] Wunderink RG, Laterre PF, Francois B, Perrotin D, Artigas A, Vidal LO, Lobo SM, Juan JS, Hwang SC, Dugernier T, LaRosa S, Wittebole X, Dhainaut JF, Doig C, Mendelson MH, Zwingelstein C, Su G, Opal S. Recombinant tissue factor pathway inhibitor in severe community-acquired pneumonia: a randomized trial. *Am. J. Respir. Crit. Care Med.,* 183(11): 1561-8,2011.

[67] Bernard GR, Ely EW, Wright TJ, Fraiz J, Stasek JE, Jr., Russell JA, Mayers I, Rosenfeld BA, Morris PE, Yan SB, Helterbrand JD. Safety and dose relationship of recombinant human activated protein C for coagulopathy in severe sepsis. *Crit. Care Med.,* 29(11): 2051-9, 2001.

[68] Abraham E, Laterre PF, Garg R, Levy H, Talwar D, Trzaskoma BL, Francois B, Guy JS, Bruckmann M, Rea-Neto A, Rossaint R, Perrotin D, Sablotzki A, Arkins N, Utterback BG, Macias WL. Drotrecogin alfa (activated) for adults with severe sepsis and a low risk of death. *N. Engl. J. Med.,* 353(13): 1332-41, 2005.

[69] Levi M, Levy M, Williams MD, Douglas I, Artigas A, Antonelli M, Wyncoll D, Janes J, Booth FV, Wang D, Sundin DP, Macias WL. Prophylactic heparin in patients with severe sepsis treated with drotrecogin alfa (activated). *Am. J. Respir. Crit. Care Med.,* 176(5): 483-90, 2007.

[70] Hartman DL BG, Helterbrand JD, Yan SB, Fisher CJ. Recombinant human activated protein C (rhAPC) improves coagulation abnormalities

associated with severe sepsis. *Intensive Care Medicine,* 24((Suppl 1)): S77, 1998.

[71] Dellinger RP, Levy MM, Carlet JM, Bion J, Parker MM, Jaeschke R, Reinhart K, Angus DC, Brun-Buisson C, Beale R, Calandra T, Dhainaut JF, Gerlach H, Harvey M, Marini JJ, Marshall J, Ranieri M, Ramsay G, Sevransky J, Thompson BT, Townsend S, Vender JS, Zimmerman JL, Vincent JL. Surviving Sepsis Campaign: international guidelines for management of severe sepsis and septic shock: 2008. *Crit. Care Med.,* 36(1): 296-327, 2008.

[72] Dhainaut JF, Laterre PF, Janes JM, Bernard GR, Artigas A, Bakker J, Riess H, Basson BR, Charpentier J, Utterback BG, Vincent JL. Drotrecogin alfa (activated) in the treatment of severe sepsis patients with multiple-organ dysfunction: data from the PROWESS trial. *Intensive Care Med.,* 29(6): 894-903, 2003.

[73] Marti-Carvajal AJ, Sola I, Lathyris D, Cardona AF. Human recombinant activated protein C for severe sepsis. *Cochrane Database Syst. Rev.,* 4): CD004388,2011.

[74] Wiedermann CJ KN. A meta-analysis of controlled trials of recombinant human activated protein C therapy in patients with sepsis. *BMC Emergency Medicine,* 5(7): 2005.

[75] Ranieri VM, Thompson BT, Barie PS, Dhainaut JF, Douglas IS, Finfer S, Gardlund B, Marshall JC, Rhodes A, Artigas A, Payen D, Tenhunen J, Al-Khalidi HR, Thompson V, Janes J, Macias WL, Vangerow B, Williams MD. Drotrecogin alfa (activated) in adults with septic shock. *N. Engl. J. Med.,* 366(22): 2055-64,2012.

[76] Wenzel RP, Edmond MB. Septic shock--evaluating another failed treatment. *N. Engl. J. Med.,* 366(22): 2122-4,2012.

[77] Esmon CT. The regulation of natural anticoagulant pathways. *Science,* 235(4794): 1348-52, 1987.

[78] Nawroth PP, Stern DM. Modulation of endothelial cell hemostatic properties by tumor necrosis factor. *J. Exp. Med.,* 163(3): 740-5, 1986.

[79] Nagato M, Okamoto K, Abe Y, Higure A, Yamaguchi K. Recombinant human soluble thrombomodulin decreases the plasma high-mobility group box-1 protein levels, whereas improving the acute liver injury and survival rates in experimental endotoxemia. *Crit. Care Med.,* 37(7): 2181-6, 2009.

[80] Iba T, Nakarai E, Takayama T, Nakajima K, Sasaoka T, Ohno Y. Combination effect of antithrombin and recombinant human soluble

thrombomodulin in a lipopolysaccharide induced rat sepsis model. *Crit. Care,* 13(6): R203, 2009.

[81] Saito H, Maruyama I, Shimazaki S, Yamamoto Y, Aikawa N, Ohno R, Hirayama A, Matsuda T, Asakura H, Nakashima M, Aoki N. Efficacy and safety of recombinant human soluble thrombomodulin (ART-123) in disseminated intravascular coagulation: results of a phase III, randomized, double-blind clinical trial. *J. Thromb. Haemost,* 5(1): 31-41, 2007.

[82] Kaul I TK, Gorelick K, Osawa Y, Hoppensteadt D, Fareed J, Vincent JL. A Randomized, Double-Blind, PlaceboControlled, Phase-2B Study to Evaluate the Safety and Efficacy of Recombinant Human Soluble Thrombomodulin, ART-123, in Patients with Sepsis and Suspected Disseminated Intravascular Coagulation. In http://www.akpamerica.com /news.htm, 2013.

[83] Kaul I. A Randomized, Double-Blind, Placebo-Controlled, Phase 3 Study to Assess the Safety and Efficacy of ART-123 in Subjects With Severe Sepsis and Coagulopathy. In http://www.clinicaltrials.gov/ct2 /show/NCT01598831?term=%22sepsis%22+AND+%22ART-123%22& rank =2, 2012.

[84] Eichacker PQ, Parent C, Kalil A, Esposito C, Cui X, Banks SM, Gerstenberger EP, Fitz Y, Danner RL, Natanson C. Risk and the efficacy of antiinflammatory agents: retrospective and confirmatory studies of sepsis. *Am. J. Respir. Crit. Care Med.,* 166(9): 1197-205, 2002.

[85] Bergmann S, Hammerschmidt S. Fibrinolysis and host response in bacterial infections. *Thromb. Haemost,* 98(3): 512-20, 2007.

[86] Zeerleder S, Hack CE, Wuillemin WA. Disseminated intravascular coagulation in sepsis. *Chest,* 128(4): 2864-75, 2005.

[87] Fourrier F. Severe sepsis, coagulation, and fibrinolysis: dead end or one way? *Crit. Care Med.,* 40(9): 2704-8, 2013.

In: Disseminated Intravascular Coagulation (DIC)   ISBN: 978-1-62948-323-8
Editor: Balwinder Singh   © 2014 Nova Science Publishers, Inc.

Chapter VII

Coagulopathy of Liver Disease versus Disseminated Intravascular Coagulation: Who is Who?

Pablo Moreno Franco MD[*1], *Jose Yataco MD*[1],
Balwinder Singh MD[2] *and Juan Canabal MD*[1]

[1]Department of Transplant Department of Transplant Critical Care Service,
Mayo Clinic, Jacksonville, Florida, US
[2]Divison of Pulmonary and Critical Care Medicine, Mayo Clinic,
Rochester, Minnesota, US

Abstract

Introduction: One of the most challenging differential diagnoses in acute care medicine is between Coagulopathy of Liver Disease (CLD) and Disseminated Intravascular Coagulation (DIC). In this chapter we contrast and compare CLD and DIC in regards to the possible etiologies,

---

[*] Corresponding Author address: Email: morenofranco.pablo@mayo.edu, Department of Transplant Critical Care Service, Tel (Critical Care): (904) 956-3298 , Fax: (904) 956-3262, Mayo Clinic , 4500 San Pablo Road, Mayo Bldg 3 North , Jacksonville, Florida 32224.

presentation, pathophysiology, diagnostic tests and management strategies.

Background: Liver disease is a broad term, but in our discussion here it refers particularly to three different entities chronic compensated cirrhosis, acute liver failure (ALF) and acute-on-chronic liver failure (ACLF). Chronic liver disease, particularly end-stage, is characterized by clinical bleeding and decreased level of most procoagulant factors with the notable exception of factor VIII and von Willebrand factor. Decreased levels of the procoagulants are, however, accompanied by decreases in levels of such naturally occurring anticoagulants as antithrombin (AT) and protein C. Coagulopathy is an essential component of the ALF syndrome and reflects the central role of the liver function in hemostasis.

Presentation: Because liver disease alters pathways of coagulation and anticoagulation, patients who have advanced disease can experience severe bleeding or thrombotic complications. History and physical examination as classically taught can help identify those patients with chronic liver disease who present with an acute decompensation. The diagnosis of ALF may be more elusive, it includes the presence of encephalopathy and coagulation abnormalities within 24 weeks of onset of acute liver disease.

Pathophysiology: The mechanisms of coagulopathy in ALF are multifactorial and include diminished synthesis of procoagulant factors, impaired anticoagulant and fibrinolytic systems, and defective function and number of platelets. Failure of the liver to remove activated procoagulants may also contribute to the development of a picture suggesting disseminated intravascular coagulation (DIC).

Diagnosis: End-organ microthrombi, if present, suggest DIC while normal ATIII, normal Factor VIII, and absence of microthrombi suggest predominant fibrinolysis. INR use in CLD is neither justified nor suitable to secure harmonization of results across clinical laboratories that use different thromboplastins for PT testing. In patients undergoing liver transplantation, and in patients with liver cirrhosis and ongoing bacterial infection, heparinase-modified thromboelastography (hep-TEG) has detected endogenous heparinoids. TEG has been used for several decades to guide transfusion goals in liver transplant centers.

Treatment: In liver disease patients, the hard-to-dye belief of correcting the abnormal traditional hemostasis tests prior to biopsy should be reconsidered. While platelet transfusion may be useful to correct severe thrombocytopenia; plasma, anti-fibrinolytic, or recombinant coagulation agents should be used with caution and decision made on an individual basis.

Conclusion: A multidisciplinary team approach is needed to appropriately diagnose and triage patients with severe coagulopathy of liver disease. Specialized testing, like factor VIII levels or TEG, may be needed to confirm the diagnosis and guide therapy. Treatment may vary, including transfusions, recombinant agents, and transplantation, depending on the clinical situation.

Keywords: Acute liver failure, chronic liver disease, coagulopathy of liver disease, disseminated intravascular coagulation, thromboelastography

Introduction

There is no debate that the care of patients with liver dysfunction is challenging. A sole medical specialty dedicated to the care of this group of patients is still a big endeavour. For the most part, a mutidisciplinary team approach may be needed for complex cases and specific scenarios. Depending on the center of care, in some instances, the Primary Care Physician will seek the assistance of the Hepatologist as well other specialties like Hematology, Nephrology, Critical Care, Infectious diseases, and Transplant Surgery. One of the most challenging differential diagnoses in acute care medicine is between Coagulopathy of Liver Disease (CLD) and Disseminated Intravascular Coagulation (DIC), especially when patients have clinical evidence of bleeding.

In this chapter, we will attempt to contrast and compare CLD and DIC with regards to the possible etiologies, presentation, pathophysiology, diagnostic tests, and management strategies.

Background

The world of coagulation is so complex and diversified that an entire medical specialty is dedicated to it. The understanding of the coagulation cascade has opened Medicine to be able to treat or prevent multiple medical problems, like hemophilias, venous thromboembolism, and coronary artery disease among others. Treatment alternatives have been put forward based on the understanding of this cascade. Chronic liver disease is perhaps the best example among diseases in Hematology as several concomitant abnormalities are observed.

Detailed description of the coagulation cascade is beyond the scope of this chapter and we assumed some basic understanding of the coagulation/anticoagulation systems.

Disseminated intravascular coagulation is the most striking manifestation of intravascular activation of the coagulation system with loss of localization. The end result is increased thrombin generation and increased fibrinolysis. It is always a complication of an underlying process that triggers a cascade of events.

The presence of these underlying processes (e.g., sepsis, trauma, malignancies) in combination with the typical laboratory abnormalities will make the clinician suspect the presence of DIC. The two clinical forms of DIC share clinical manifestations, but differ in the duration and the extension of the laboratory abnormalities.

Acute DIC develops shortly after the offending event with excessive thrombin generation, massive consumption of coagulation factors and platelets, and microthrombis formation. Chronic DIC patients have compensatory mechanisms activated that replenish the depleted coagulation factors and platelets to a certain degree. As a consequence, they could be asymptomatic or may have some minor skin and mucosal bleeding.

Liver disease is a broad term, but in our discussion here it refers particularly to three different entities: chronic compensated cirrhosis (sometimes labeled End Stage Liver Disease, ESLD), acute liver failure (ALF), and acute-on-chronic liver failure (ACLF), sometimes refered to as "decompensated" liver failure. Chronic compensated cirrhotic patients, for the most part, have no signs of clinically significant bleeding. It is traditionally understood that patients with liver disease have a complex coagulation profile that points in the direction of hypocoagulable state. This is not what is commonly seen in practice and, in fact, many patients do not have any clinical evidence of bleeding or thrombosis.

This is contrary to common teaching assumptions based on their laboratory data. The most frequently used tests for screening and monitoring (PT, PTT, INR, and Platelet count) do not do justice to the complexity of the disease. In industrialized nations, these tests are widely available and very commonly used. There is variability in the testing results, but for the most part, the clinicians seem to be very comfortable relying on them. Of note, these tests do not say a thing about the global in vivo coagulation state of the patient. More "sophisticated" tests that attempt to measure *global hemostasis* may not be widely available at many centers.

Tests like Thrombin Generation Test (TGT), Thromboelastogram (TEG), and clot wave form analysis (APTT WA) have their particular pitfalls [34] and not all clinicians are educated in their use and interpretation. This makes it difficult to use them as holy grails in the evaluation of the coagulopathic patient but certainly, if available, may help direct prophylaxis/treatment of replacement products in this population.

In patients with chronic compensated cirrhosis, there is liver dysfunction and thus all pro-coagulants synthetized by the liver (antithombin, prothrombin [Factor II], fibrinogen, plasminogen, antithrombin III, factors V, VII, X, XI, XII and XIII) will be low. Anti-coagulants like Protein C and S are also low. [27, 28, 54] ALF or ACLF could be characterized by clinical bleeding and decreased level of most procoagulant factors with the notable exception of factor VIII and von Willebrand factor. [50] Decreased levels of the procoagulants are, however, accompanied by decreases in levels of such naturally occurring anticoagulants as antithrombin (AT) and protein C. [50] Coagulopathy is an essential component of the ALF syndrome and reflects the central role of the liver function in hemostasis. [33]

Clinical Presentation

The clinical manifestations of DIC include bleeding from catheter sites, wounds, drains, mucosal surfaces, gastrointestinal tract, lungs, and Central Nervous System (CNS). Organ dysfunction includes acute renal failure, hepatic dysfunction with jaundice and elevated liver enzymes, changes in mental status with or without focal findings and pulmonary manifestation with dyspnea, hypoxemia, hemoptysis, and Acute Respiratory Distress Syndrome (ARDS).

The chronic form of DIC, usually triggered by solid malignant tumors, is more likely to present with thrombotic events that include deep vein thrombosis, arterial thrombosis, and strokes.

Liver disease in the forms of ALF, compensated chronic liver disease, and decompensated chronic liver disease can mimick the laboratory findings and clinical manifestations of DIC. The clinical scenario and a few diagnostic laboratory tests may help achieve a more precise diagnosis.

Clinically, the chronic stable cirrhotic patient may have easy bruising or mucocutaneous manifestations particularly blamed on the commonly found thrombocytopenia. Other commonly abnormal tests are elevated PTT and INR triggering the thought of a bleeding-prone patient. In fact, it is abnormalities in fibrinogen that make the PTT/INR become elevated, falsely suggesting hypocoagulability in these patients.

The myth that liver patients are protected from thrombotic complications has been put to rest. Patients with compensated or decompensated liver cirrhosis, that are less than 45 years old, have an increased risk of Venous Thromboembolism (VTE). [57] Mesenteric and Portal Venous thrombosis have been reported to be about 15% in patients awaiting liver transplant. [44, 50] This patient population is also thought to be at greater risk of bleeding complications like variceal bleeding, reported to be as high as 15% per year. [8] So, this creates a dicotomy, how is it that a patient with low platelets, prolonged PTT, and prolonged INR can bleed but also form clot? As elegantly written by *Tripodi* et al., there is a new fragile balance in the pro-coagulant/anti-coagulant system in chronic liver disease. [50] This balance can be easily disturbed by events like infections, trauma, and surgery, making the diagnosis of CLD and/or DIC even more difficult.

DIC is a clinicopathologic diagnosis that has features of clinical bleeding and thrombosis. [3] This is potentially the source of confusion as it does not rely solely on laboratory tests where most of them are very similar to the ones found on liver patients (specially the "decompensated" cirrhotics). Common laboratory abnormalities in DIC are: low platelet count, prolonged PT, prolonged thombin time (TT), prolonged PTT, decreased fibrinogen and elevated levels of fibrinogen degradation products (FDP). Fibrinolysis is present in DIC with elevated prothrombin fragments 1+2 (F1 + 2), thombin-antithrombin complexes (TAT). Some authors have demonstrated that in fact DIC is not part of the coagulopathy of stable cirrhotic patient as there are not demonstrable changes in FDP or F1+2. [3]. Now, in patients with ACLF were there can be a trigger can elicit a fibrinolytic response elevating such parameters. Infection, among other triggers can alter that fragile balance towards fibrinolisys making the patient more susceptible to bleeding. In fact, an entity named accelerated intravascular coagulation and fibrinolysis (AICF) wich is very similar to DIC has been found in ~30% of patients with moderate to severe liver failure and not in chronic compensated cirrhotics. [8]

ALF is the development of severe liver dysfunction with hepatic encephalopathy and coagulopathy in an individual without cirrhosis or preexisting liver disease. Laboratory findings include prolonged prothrombin time with INR ≥ 1.5 (must be present), minimal or no prolongation of PTT, thrombocytopenia, and usually normal fibrinogen levels. The differentation with DIC is for the most part simple, with ALF having marked elevation in aminotransferance, bilirrubin, and ammonia levels. The clinical manifestations of ALF are initially nonspecific with malaise, lethargy, nausea/vomiting, and pruritus followed by more particular manifestations of liver disease like progressive hepatic encephalopathy, jaundice, and ascitis. The prolonged prothrombin time and thrombocytopenia in ALF, along with the decline in both procoagulant and anticoagulant factors, cause a disturbance in the coagulation homeostasis that is complex and heterogenous. [2, 22] Based on TEG, 45% of patients with ALF have a normal coagulable state, 20% have a hypocoagulable state, and 35% are hypercoagulable. [2]

Patients with chronic liver disease have profound abnormalities in the coagulation system, with a rebalanced hemostatic state that is precarious and unhealthy compared to normal individuals. This restored balance of homeostasis may easily shift to either hypo or hypercoagulability under precipitating circumstances like infections, toxins, and ischemia.

Chronic liver disease may be present for years without diagnosis and patients with liver disease could be asymptomatic or minimally symptomatic until a moment of acute decompensation with a myriad of manifestations. In the past, autopsy series reported cirrhosis in up to 30-40% of cases. [12] Those undiagnosed individuals, unaware of their chronic liver disease can present with bleeding and thrombotic complications in addition to multiple organ failure very similar to those present in disseminated intravascular coagulation.

The suspicion for underlying chronic liver disease has to start with a detailed history and physical exam. The past medical history should focus on history of alcohol consumption, viral hepatitis, use of illicit drugs, history of transfusions, and history of systemic, autoinmmune, or congenital diseases. They usually have a long time history of fatigue, weight loss, peripheral edema, easy bruising, pruritus, ascites, and mild cognitive deficits.

A number of physical findings can be present in chronic liver disease. [16, 25] The skin examination can reveal:

- Jaundice, usually detectable when bilirrubin level is above 2.5 mg/dl
- Palmar erythema, increased speckled mottling pattern of the palm, on the thenar and hypothenar eminences of the palm
- Nail changes, horizontal white bands alteranting with normal color, nonspecific finding
- Telangiectasias, mostly distributed on the trunk, face and upper limbs. The density and size of these spider angiomata correlate with the severity of liver disease
- Clubbing and hypertrophic osteoarthropathy
- Dupuytren's contracture, wich results from thickening and shortening of the palmar fascia

Other physical findings in liver disease include:

- Splenomegaly
- Hepatomegaly, although cirrhosis can also have normal or small liver size
- Ascites
- Caput Medusae
- Gynecomastia and testicular atrophy
- Asterixis

Patients with very advanced chronic liver disease or decompensated cirrhosis have serious disarrangements of hemostasis. A severe decrease in most of the factors involved in the coagulation system, procoagulants, anticoagulants and thrombocytopenia create a frail situation with active bleeding and sometimes thrombosis/organ dysfunction that resembles DIC. Patients can present with mucosal bleed, epistaxis, purpura, easy bruising and spontaneous bleed from drains and catheters.

More serious manifestation of bleed can take place in the lungs, gastrointestinal tract or central nervous system, sometimes with catastrophic consequences.

Pathophysiology

Chronic liver disease causes a very complex change in the coagulation system that is not detected by routine hemostatic tests like platelet count and measurement of PT/PTT.

In normal individuals with acute illness, including DIC, they may indicate a propensity for spontaneous bleeds. This is not the case for patients with chronic liver disease in which laboratory and clinical evidence indicate that the hemostatic system is in a "rebalance" status with changes in procoagulant factors, anticoagulant factors, platelets and fibrynolysis. [19, 20, 29, 41, 53]

Viral infections, ETOH, NASH, Wilson's, Drug toxicity
Sepsis Post-surgical Uncontrolled bleeding
Trauma Malignancy Obstetric complications
CLD
AICF
DIC
Encephalopathy Jaundice
ALF
Stigmata of chronic liver disease
CLF
ACLF
Presentation
Bleeding
Decreased production of nonendothelial derived coagulation factors
Rebalanced coagulation
Pathophysiology
Decreased liver synthesized anticoagulant proteins
Thrombosis
Thrombocytopenia
Fibrinolysis
Usually elevated Maybe NL or Decreased
VIII
Usually elevated
Ammonia
Tests
To guide therapy
TEG
Vitamin K
Treatment
Transfusions
If bleeding
Abnormal TEG
Platelets If < 10-20K or < 50K pre-procedure
DDAVP
Ultimately OLT maybe required
Treat or control underlying cause
FFP
Cryoprecipitate
If concomitant renal dysfunction
Corrects coagulopathy in days - weeks
Shortly after insult
Acute DIC
AKI, ARDS, Increased LFTs
Presentation
Chronic DIC
Compensatory mechanisms to replenish coagulation factors and platelets
Pathophysiology
Excessive thrombing generation
Massive Consumption of coagulation factors and platelets
Microthrombus formation
VIII
Low
Tests
Ammonia
NL
Treatment
Do not transfuse if no bleed
Except: PLT if < 10-20K
Expert opinion
Heparin
No RCT
FFP?
Treatment of underlying cause
Unless: DVT Arterial thrombosis Purpura fulminans Arterial ischemia

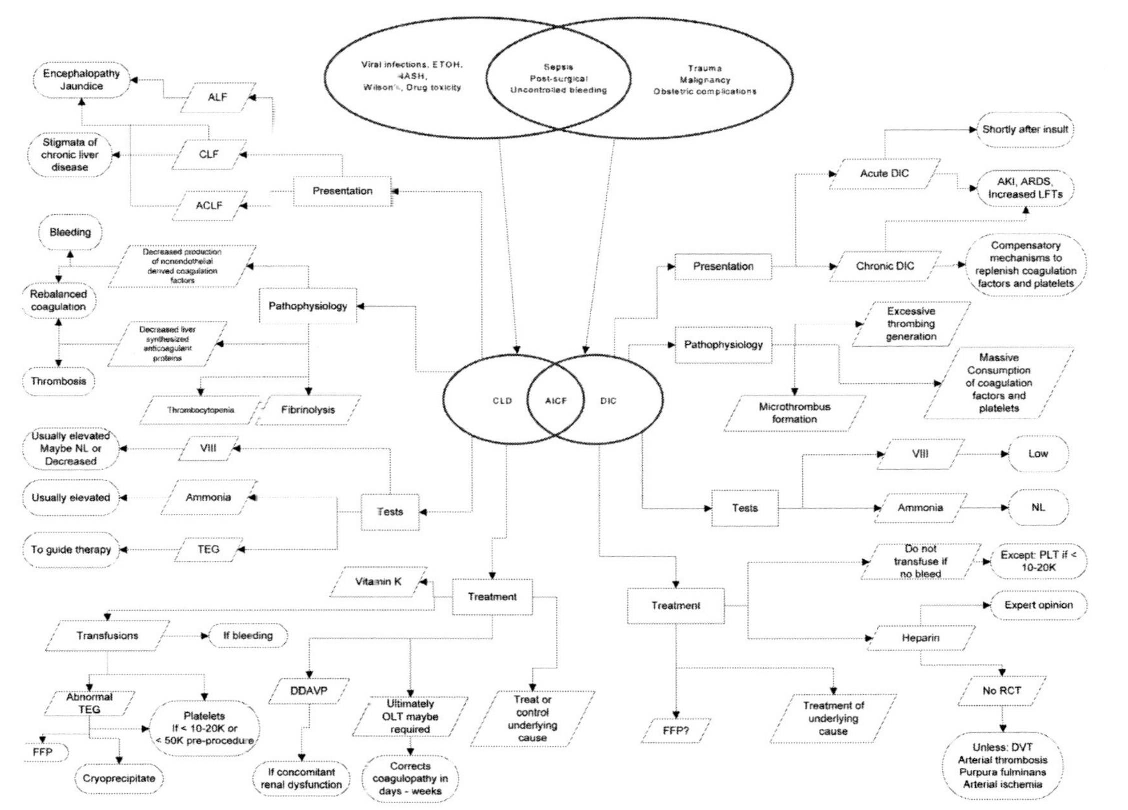

Figure 1.

Table 1.

	DIC	ALF	CLF	ACLF
Etiology	Sepsis, trauma, post-surgical, obstetric complications, malignancy, others	Tylenol overdose, Viral infection, ETOH, Wilsons, Drugs, others	Chronic Viral Hepatitis, ETOH, NASH, Wilsons, Others	Superimposed infection, superimposed medication toxicity, ischemic insult, drug toxicity, surgeries, others
Physical exam	Variable	Encephalopathy, +/- jaundice	Stigmata of chronic liver disease	Stigmata of chronic liver disease may be present
Signs of clinical bleeding	plus/minus	plus/minus	plus/minus	plus/minus
Manifestations	AKI, hepatic dysfunction with jaundice and elevated liver enzymes, hypoxemia, hemoptysis and ARDS	Initially malaise, lethargy, nausea/vomiting, pruritus followed by hepatic encephalopathy, jaundice and (rarely) ascitis	Easy bruising, mucocutaneous manifestations, gastrointestinal bleed	Combination of acute and chronic manifestations
Hb	Variable	Variable	Usually low	Usually low
Peripheral Smear	may have schistozytes	Variable	macrocytosis, acanthocytes and target cells	Variable
PT	Prolonged	Usually prolonged	Nl/prolonged	NL or Prolonged in AICF
INR	Prolonged	Prolonged ≥ 1.5 (must be present)	Nl/prolonged	NL or Prolonged in AICF
PTT	Prolonged	plus/minus	Variable	Variable
Platelet count	Low	Variable	Low	Low
Factor VIII	Low	Usually elevated if low suggests DIC	NL/low	Nl/low
Von Willenbrand	NL to high	NL to low	Nl-very high	NL/low
ADAMTS 13	Low	Unknown	Decreased	Decreased
ATIII	Decreased	Decreased	NL/low	Nl/low
Fibrinogen	Decreased	Usually normal	Low or normal fibrinogen by immunologic assays; and reduced fibrinogen in functional assays	Nl/low
Fibrinogen Degradation Products	Elevated	Variable	Variable	Elevated in AICF
TEG	Fibrinolysis	45% normal, 20% hypocoagulable, 35% hypercoagulable	Normal to increased R+K time, decreased MA and angle.	Fibrinolysis in AICF
TAFI	Activated	Decreased	Decreased	Unknown
PAI-1	Decreased	Depressed in severe liver failure	Increased	Depressed in severe liver failure

	DIC	ALF	CLF	ACLF
Prothrombin fragments 1+2	Elevated	Unknown	Not significantly different than normal controls	Elevated in AICF
Thrombin-AT complexes	Present	Increase	Not significantly different than normal controls	
Protein C	Low	Low	NL/low	Nl/low
Protein S	Low	Low	Nl/low	Nl/low
Aminotransferases	Nl/slightly elevated	Marked elevation	Variable	Usually elevated
Bilirrubins	Nl/slightly elevated	Nl/Elevated	Usually elevated, depends on etiology	Usually elevated
Ammonia levels	NL	Elevated	Variable	Variable
Glucose level	Variable	Nl to decrease	Variable	Variable
Risk of venous thrombosis	Sometimes in chronic DIC usually in setting of solid organ tumor (i.e., DVT)	Rare	Yes (i.e., DVT, PVT, MVT)	Yes (i.e., DVT, PVT, MVT)
Arterial thrombosis	Sometimes in chronic DIC usually in setting of solid organ tumor (i.e., stroke)	Rare	Rare	Rare
Risk of clinical significant bleed	Yes (i.e., venipuncture site, wounds, drains, mucosal surfaces, gastrointestinal tract, lungs and CNS)	Yes (i.e., venipuncture sites, CNS)	Yes (i.e., variceal)	Yes (i.e., variceal)

ACLF: Acute on chronic liver failure; AICF: Accelerated intravascular coagulation and fibrinolysis; ALF: Acute liver failure; AT: antithrombin; ATIII: antithrombin III; CLD: Coagulopathy of liver disease; CLF: Chronic liver failure; DIC: Disseminated Intravascular Coagulation; DVT: deep venous thrombosis; INR: International Normalized Ratio; MVT: mesenteric vein thrombosis; NL: Normal; PT: Prothrombin Time; PTT: partial thromboplastin time; PVT: portal vein thrombosis; TT: thromboblastin time

Coagulation Factors

The synthetic function of the liver becomes significantly impaired with progression of liver disease. When this occurs, decreased production of non-endothelial cell derived procoagulation factors (FII, FV, FVII, FIX, FX, FXI, FXII, and fibrinogen) disturbs homeostasis in the direction of hypocoagulability. [20, 52] A simultaneous and parallel change occurs in the liver-synthesized anticoagulant proteins C, protein S, and AT III, rebalancing the coagulation system.[19, 23, 50]

Besides the liver-derived changes in the levels of procoagulants and anticoagulants, many other alterations in the haemostatic system take place to generate a new rebalance state (table 1).

Platelet Level and Function

Thrombocytopenia is almost universal with the progression of liver disease. The mechanism of thrombocytopenia is multifactorial due to a combination of hypersplenism, bone marrow depression and change in thrombopoietin metabolism. [37] However, patients with liver disease very commonly have very high levels of von Willebrand factor, which may restore platelet adhesion properties to the subendothelium at sites of vascular injury. [18] Furthermore, levels of ADAMTS 13 are reduced in cirrhosis, this may further contribute to the restoration of platelet function. [50]

Using an assay that resembles in vivo thrombin generation, a platelet count of 56,000/microL has been demonstrated to produce enough thrombin at a level equivalent to the lower limit of the normal range in healthy subjects. [51]

Fibrinolysis

After deposition of fibrin within the vascular system, a tightly regulated process of fibrinolysis converts the proenzyme plasminogen into the active enzyme plasmin, in charge of degrading fibrin. Evidence of increased fibrinolysis has been reported in a high percentage of patients with liver disease in parallel to the degree of liver dysfunction. [17] Cirrhotic patients have some laboratory findings that favor hyperfibrinolysis: increased levels of TPA, reduced levels of plasmin inhibitor and reduced levels of TAFI. Simultaneously, they also have changes that cause hypofibrinolysis: reduced plasminogen levels and increased levels of PAI (Plasminogen activator inhibitor). [21] Therefore, the balance of fibrinolysis in compensated liver disease is probably restored by the parallel changes in profibrinolitic and antifibrinolitic drivers. However, an acute event causing decompensation of liver disease (i.e., sepsis, trauma, and toxins) can perturbate this fine balance triggering hyperfibrinolysis with hemorrhage or hypofibrinolysis with thrombosis.

Under these circumstances, it could be very difficult to differentiate clinically the presentation of decompensated chronic liver disease from the syndrome of disseminated intravascular coagulation that follows an acute trigger.

Diagnostic Tests

There is no single test that can make the diagnosis of DIC. Likewise, there is no single test that can make the diagnosis of CLD. Tests commonly used as a starting point for diagnosis include: hemoglobin level, platelet count, and blood smear analysis. Specialized coagulation laboratories that include PT, aPTT, TT, TEG, FDP, and certain coagulation factor levels may generate the highest diagnostic yiels. There may also be some value to measuring liver function tests, particularly bilirubin level, albumin level, glucose level and degree of elevation as well as trend of transaminases.

Anemia and several morphologic changes, including macrocytosis, acanthocytes, and target cells, can be seen in patients with liver disease and hypersplenism. These changes are usually secondary to the combination of abnormal lipid metabolism, excess cholesterol content in the outer leaflet of the RBC membrane, and deformation stress during transit through splenic microcirculation. [55]

Thrombocytopenia is the most common and first of the abnormal hematologic indices to occur in patients with cirrhosis, followed by leukopenia and anemia. [39] Patients with liver disease and thrombocytopenia have serum thrombopoietin concentration higher than normal controls. [11] In the liver patients, the number of circulating platelets and the serum levels of thrombopoietin are inversely correlated with the size of the spleen, suggesting that thrombopoietin, although normally produced, might be turned over in platelets sequestrated in the spleen. [11]

Leukopenia is also a frequent laboratory finding in coagulopathy of liver disease. A combination of leukopenia and thrombocytopenia at baseline predict increased morbidity and mortality. [39]

Historically, PT/INR has been used in patients with chronic liver disease as part of prognostic indices such as Child-Pugh score and model for end-stage-liver-disease score (MELD). But several studies have shown that PT, INR, and aPTT are not good predictors of gastrointestinal or post-procedural bleeding. [42, 52] The other problem is that INR has not been validated in patients with cirrhosis. INR use in CLD is neither justified or suitable to secure harmonization of results across clinical laboratories that use different thromboplastins for PT testing. [49] PT and PTT are designed to be sensitive to procoagulant proteins, but not to anticoagulant proteins that are also decreased in liver disease. The obvious conclusion is that the value of trying to correct these parameters to specific "goals" borrowed from other patient populations is uncertain. Therefore, the clinician should consider if transfusion of expensive and potentially harmful blood products or procoagulant factors is really indicated, either by clinical scenario of ongoing bleeding or TEG abnormalities.

With the exception of tPA and PAI-1, all fibrinolytic and antifibrinolytic proteins are synthesized in the liver. [20] When measuring PAI-1 it has been found to be elevated in patients with chronic liver disease, but depressed in severe liver failure. [4] Decreased hepatic clearance of tPA and reduced synthesis of alfa2 anti-plasmin and thrombin activatable fibrinolysis inhibitor (TAFI) favor both an increase in circulating plasmin and a hyperfibrinolytic state in cirrhosis.

FDP is one of the most sensitive tests for DIC. Unfortunately, this test may not be helpful to differentiate from CLD due to impaired hepatic clearance. What is important to know is that in CLD, compared to DIC, these parameters do not change rapidly. End-organ microthrombi, if present, suggest DIC, while normal ATIII, normal Factor VIII, and absence of microthrombi suggests predominant fibrinolysis. [33] Dysfibrinogenemia has been reported in up to 75% of patients with chronic liver disease, cirrhosis, and ALF. Characteristic laboratory finding of dysfibrinogenemia include elevated PT, aPTT or TT; low or normal fibrinogen by immunologic assays; and reduced fibrinogen in functional assays. Even in the presence of these abnormalities, the role of dysfibrinogenemia as a contributing factor to bleeding in liver disease patients is not clearly established.

Accelerated intravascular coagulation and fibrinolysis (AICF) has been detected in up to 30% of cirrhotics, depending on the degree of liver failure. [5, 43] This diagnosis would require the use of highly sensitive tests, such as prothrombin fragment 1+2 (a marker of in vivo thrombin generation), D-Dimer (a product of thrombin and plasmin activation), high-molecular-weight fibrin/fibrinogen complexes, or soluble fibrin. [8] AICF probably results from the formation of a fibrin clot that is more susceptible to plasmin degradation because of elevated tPA levels or the presence of dysfibrinogenemia. [8] AICF seems to occur predominantly in patients who have moderate-to-severe liver failure, but is not detected in compensated patients. [53]

Hyperfibrinolysis has been associated closely with the degree of liver failure and ascites and constitutes a further risk, in adition to variceal size, in predicting gastrointestinal bleeding. [56] As a consequence of hyperfibrinolysis, clotting activation maybe delayed because of the consumption of clotting factors and inhibition of fibrin polymerization. [31] Hyperfibrinolysis also reduces platelet adhesion and aggregation by degradation of von Willebrand's factor and fibrinogen platelet receptors (glycoprotein Ib and IIb/IIIa). [46] Hyperfibrinolysis may provoke clot lysis by inducing platelet disaggregation and disruption of the hemostatic plug. [26]Hyperfibrinolysis may delay primary hemostasis or clotting activation or induce disruption of the hemostatic plug, thereby aggravating variceal bleeding and increasing the likelihood of recurrence. [46]

For many years TEG has been used by anesthesiologists and intensivists in patients with ESLD, ALF, and ACLF who present with bleeding disorders or during the perioperative period. TEG allows in-vitro analysis of the interactive dynamic coagulation processes, from initial clotting cascade and platelet interaction to clot strengthening and fibrinolysis. It has also been successfully used to detect hypercoagulable states and offers a valid alternative to standard tests. In patients undergoing liver transplantation, and in patients with liver cirrhosis and ongoing bacterial infection, heparinase-modified thromboelastography (hep-TEG) has detected endogenous heparinoids. [58] Until recently the role of TEG in non-transplant related liver resections had not been well characterized. An Italian group conducted a very detailed study to characterize the coagulation profiles of this patients based on TEG. They found TEG evidence of normocoagulability in the liver resection group, despite early increase in INR and aPTT and reduction in PLTs, fibrinogen, and ATIII in all patients studied. [7] Prior studies had also shown the important role of TEG in evaluating coagulation and platelet function [47] and in guiding the treatment depending on what particular parameter is altered. [45] Therefore, one of the most valuable tests to assess coagulopathy and guide therapy in CLD is TEG.

Treatment

The main concept here is that the clinician should not treat laboratory abnormalities that do not translate as clinically significant syndromes. For example a patient with mild thrombocytopenia and elevated INR, who has minor mucosal bleeding, may not require expensive and risky transfusions.

In liver disease patients, the hard-to-dye belief of correcting the abnormal traditional hemostasis tests prior to liver biopsy should be reconsidered. This is an area of debate, but the majority of providers agree that patients should avoid drugs that may alter coagulation or platelet function, platelet count should be above 50,000, and even if the prothrombin time is elevated by more than three seconds, the risk of bleeding is minimal. Patients who have greater abnormalities of coagulation may receive fresh frozen plasma (FFP) or platelet transfusions before the procedure. [54] The caveat here is that there is no evidence to determine that specific "goals" need to be met. Given risk/costs related to these transfusions, an intermediate approach directed to transfuse just before and even during the procedure itself, may be a safer and better blood product management strategy.

Oral vitamin K and bile salts are sufficient for treatment of mild vitamin K deficiency. Intramuscular or intravenous administration of vitamin K (5mg/d) is effective in correcting PT within 24-48 hours. [13] Due to concerns with cost and risk of anaphylaxis associated with parenteral formulations, the oral route is usually preferred. Many practitioners give 10mg of vitamin K orally, unless there is need for expedited treatment with parenteral routes. In those cases the subcutaneous route is preferred, based on reported cases of anaphylaxis with intravenous administration. [10]

1-deamino-8-D-Arginine-vasopressin (DDAVP) is frequently prescribed in patients with CLD who concomitantly have renal dysfunction. DDAVP is a synthetic analog of vasopressin that acts by stimulating the release of molecular weight multimers of von Willebrand factor from endothelial cells, although other mechanisms have also been suggested. [59] It is administered intravenously at a dose of 0.3 micrograms/Kg over 30 minutes. [15] Bleeding times improve in about one hour and the effect lasts up to eight hours. [30]

FFP is perhaps too commonly used to correct INR in patients with liver disease. FFP is certainly a suitable agent for the correction of multiple coagulation defects in patients with liver disease because it contains all coagulation factors and inhibitors present in blood. [13] When the indication is correct, for example a bleeding patient with an abnormal TEG, it can be a life saving therapy. Risks commonly associated with FFP include transfusion-related acute lung injury, transfusion-associated circulatory overload, and allergic or anaphylactic reactions. Other less common risks include transmission of infections, febrile nonhemolytic transfusion reactions, red blood cell alloimmunization, and hemolytic transfusion reactions. [36]

Platelet transfusion is required for severe thrombocytopenia. In practice, platelet transfusions are commonly seen before procedures if the platelet count is less than 50 thousand. But platelet transfusions have been identified as an independent risk factor for adverse post-operative outcomes after liver transplantation. [6] The same group also reported decreased survival of liver transplantation patients as a function of platelet transfusions due to higher rates of ALI or ARDS. [38]

Since cryoprecipitate contains both fibrinogen and factors VIII and XIII, its use is rarely necessary because of the high level of factor VIII in cirrhosis. The usual indication for transfusion in this patient population is hypofibrinogenemia or severe fibrinolysis that results in selective destruction of factor VIII. Transfusion of 1 unit of cryoprecipitate containing 300 mg of fibrinogen increases the fibrinogen level approximately 10 mg/dl in a patient weighting 60 Kg. The half life of fibrinogen is approximately 3-4 days, and repeated transfusions of cryoprecipitate are necessary to supplement the loss. [13] During liver transplantation trans-p-aminoacetyl-cyclohexanecarboxylic acid has been used without complications and E-aminocaproic acid has proved to be very effective in treating fibrinolysis. [14]

Thrombopeitin receptor agonists have been studied in an attempt to improve platelet count before procedures and try to avoid platelet transfusions. Eltrombopag has been coparted to placebo and there is evidence that its use increased platelet count and drecreased the amount of platelet transfusions. But most importantly there was no significant difference between the two groups in terms of bleeding episodes of WHO 2 or higher. Futhermore, Eltrombopag was associated with an increased incidence of portal-vein thrombosis. [1]

Ultimately liver transplantation may be the only answer to improve the condition of a patient with advanced liver disease who happens to present with coagulopathy as one of many other organ dysfunctions. Ironically, reperfusion of the grafted liver is also intitially associated with severe coagulopathy; dilutional coagulopathy from the influx of preservation solution, heparin effect from the release of heparin or heparin-like substances from the donor hepatocytes, explosive fibrinolysis by the release of tPA from donor liver, and inhibition of coagulation by other unknown substances. The cause of the pathological coagulation is determined by comparing the thromboelastography results of whole blood, blood treated with protamine sulfate, and blood treated with E-aminocaproid acid. [14] If heparin effect persists 30 minutes after reperfusion, it is treated with 25 to 50 mg of protamine sulfate. E-aminocaproic acid (250-500 mg, single dose) is administered to treat fibrinolysis (fibrinolysis time <60 minutes) in approximately 60% of patients. [13] Fortunately, severe coagulopathy improves gradually during the neohepatic stage unless major surgical bleeding continues. The coagulation profile (PT, aPTT, and platelet count) improves gradually and normalized 2-4 weeks after transplantation.

Recent data from Findlay and colleagues show that, compared to a historical control, a recent cohort of patient undergoing liver transplantation had significantly fewer perioperative allogeneic red blood cell transfusions, intraoperative autotransfusions, and transfusions of other blood products. [9] Importantly, there was no significant change in morbidity or mortality and the rate of reoperations decreased significantly. The overall patient survival at one and five years was not significantly altered; however, graft survival at one year was significantly higher in the recent cohort. The authors attribute the decrease in transfusion requirements primarily to changes in surgical technique without a significant alteration in transfusion triggers. Interestingly, since that cohort, there has been a tendency to alterations in transfusion triggers directed to minimize transfusions. We will stay tuned for the outcomes of these changes.

While platelet transfusion may be useful to correct severe thrombocytopenia; plasma, anti-fibrinolytic, or recombinant coagulation agents should be used with caution and decision made on an individual basis. [48] Essentially, careful consideration based on patients' clinical status and many different static and dynamic coagulation tests is key to the successful treatment of CLD.

The treatment of DIC is addressed in other chapters in detail, but as it pertains to the patient with liver disease it remains controversial because of the complexity of the clinical picture. Cryoprecipitate can be administered to increase the fibrinogen level, but it may accelerate coagulation. The use of heparin with the additional administration of ATIII containing FFP appears to be effective.[40] However, heparin is not recommended unless a definite diagnosis is made. Most clinicians implement replacement therapy using FFP and platelets, with or without judicious use of heparin (<5,000U). [13]

A very complex, although uncommon, scenario appears when a patient with CLD appears to be volume overloaded and has either a bleeding complication like hemotysis or needs to be taken for an invasive procedure. In such situations the use of exchange plasmapheresis can become a life saving intervention. Essentially, the procedure is done to accomplish isovolumetric removal and transfusion of FFP. Exchange plasmapheresis allows the transfusion of large amounts of FFP in ALF. [32]

Another therapeutic option that has been under intense scrutiny is the use of clotting factor concentrates. There is an extensive list of clotting factor concentrates available in the US. Some of them represent single factor concentrates, Factor VIIa for example, while others have multiple factors like Prothrombin Complex Concentrates (PCC) that contain II, VII, IX and X. Furthermore, there are some available compounds with Activated Prothrombin Complex Concentrates. These products are approved by the FDA to be used for congenital bleeding disorders, but there are no clear indications for patients with CLD. Also there are some concerns of its efficacy and anecdotal reports of thrombosis following its administration. [24, 35]

Conclusion

A multidisciplinary team approach is needed to appropriately diagnose and triage patients with severe coagulopathy of liver disease. Medical history and physical examination continue to be a very important tool to help with this differential diagnosis. Specialized testing, like TEG, interpreted by a well-versed clinician may be needed to confirm the diagnosis and guide therapy, especially in very critically ill patients awating transplantation and peri-operatively. Treatment of CLD may include transfusions, recombinant agents, or transplantation depending on the clinical situation. The most determinant factor when evaluating treatment is a very detailed clininical decision-making process to avoid over-correction and exposing the patient to the side effect of blood product transfusions when they may not be necessary.

References

[1]   Afdhal NH, Giannini EG, Tayyab G, Mohsin A, Lee JW, Andriulli A, et al. Eltrombopag before procedures in patients with cirrhosis and thrombocytopenia. *N Engl J Med*. 2012 Aug 23;367(8):716-24.

[2]   Agarwal B, Wright G, Gatt A, Riddell A, Vemala V, Mallett S, et al. Evaluation of coagulation abnormalities in acute liver failure. *J Hepatol*. 2012 Oct;57(4):780-6.

[3]   Ben-Ari Z, Osman E, Hutton RA, Burroughs AK. Disseminated intravascular coagulation in liver cirrhosis: fact or fiction? *Am J Gastroenterol*. 1999 Oct;94(10):2977-82.

[4]   Boks AL, Brommer EJ, Schalm SW, Van Vliet HH. Hemostasis and fibrinolysis in severe liver failure and their relation to hemorrhage. *Hepatology*. 1986 Jan-Feb;6(1):79-86.

[5]   Caldwell SH, Hoffman M, Lisman T, Macik BG, Northup PG, Reddy KR, et al. Coagulation disorders and hemostasis in liver disease: pathophysiology and critical assessment of current management. *Hepatology*. 2006 Oct;44(4):1039-46.

[6]   de Boer MT, Christensen MC, Asmussen M, van der Hilst CS, Hendriks HG, Slooff MJ, et al. The impact of intraoperative transfusion of platelets and red blood cells on survival after liver transplantation. *Anesth Analg*. 2008 Jan;106(1):32-44, table of contents.

[7]   De Pietri L, Montalti R, Begliomini B, Scaglioni G, Marconi G, Reggiani A, et al. Thromboelastographic changes in liver and pancreatic cancer surgery: hypercoagulability, hypocoagulability or normocoagulability? *Eur J Anaesthesiol*. 2010 Jul;27(7):608-16.

[8]   Ferro D, Celestini A, Violi F. Hyperfibrinolysis in liver disease. *Clin Liver Dis*. 2009 Feb;13(1):21-31.

[9]   Findlay JY, Long TR, Joyner MJ, Heimbach JK, Wass CT. Changes in transfusion practice over time in adult patients undergoing liver transplantation. *J Cardiothorac Vasc Anesth*. 2013 Feb;27(1):41-5.

[10] Fiore LD, Scola MA, Cantillon CE, Brophy MT. Anaphylactoid reactions to vitamin K. *J Thromb Thrombolysis*. 2001 Apr;11(2):175-83.

[11] Freni MA, Spadaro A, Ajello A, Barbaro E, Scaffidi M, Alessi N, et al. Serum thrombopoietin in chronic liver disease: Relation to severity of the disease and spleen size. *Hepato-Gastroenterol*. 2002 Sep-Oct;49(47):1382-5.

[12] Haellen J, Norden J. Liver Cirrhosis Unsuspected during Life. A Series of 79 Cases. *J Chronic Dis*. 1964 Oct;17:951-8.

[13] Kang Y. Coagulopathies in hepatic disease. *Liver Transpl*. 2000 Jul(4 Suppl 1):S72-5.

[14] Kang Y, Lewis JH, Navalgund A, Russell MW, Bontempo FA, Niren LS, et al. Epsilon-Aminocaproic Acid for Treatment of Fibrinolysis during Liver-Transplantation. *Anesthesiology*. 1987 Jun;66(6):766-73.

[15] Kaw D, Malhotra D. Platelet dysfunction and end-stage renal disease. *Semin Dial*. 2006 Jul-Aug;19(4):317-22.

[16] LeBlond RF, DeGowin RL, Brown DD. DeGowin's diagnostic examination. 9th ed. New York: McGraw-Hill Medical; 2009.

[17] Leebeek FW, Kluft C, Knot EA, de Maat MP, Wilson JH. A shift in balance between profibrinolytic and antifibrinolytic factors causes

enhanced fibrinolysis in cirrhosis. *Gastroenterology.* 1991 Nov;101(5):1382-90.

[18] Lisman T, Bongers TN, Adelmeijer J, Janssen HL, de Maat MP, de Groot PG, et al. Elevated levels of von Willebrand Factor in cirrhosis support platelet adhesion despite reduced functional capacity. *Hepatology.* 2006 Jul;44(1):53-61.

[19] Lisman T, Caldwell SH, Burroughs AK, Northup PG, Senzolo M, Stravitz RT, et al. Hemostasis and thrombosis in patients with liver disease: the ups and downs. *J Hepatol.* 2010 Aug;53(2):362-71.

[20] Lisman T, Leebeek FW. Hemostatic alterations in liver disease: a review on pathophysiology, clinical consequences, and treatment. *Dig Surg.* 2007;24(4):250-8.

[21] Lisman T, Leebeek FW, Mosnier LO, Bouma BN, Meijers JC, Janssen HL, et al. Thrombin-activatable fibrinolysis inhibitor deficiency in cirrhosis is not associated with increased plasma fibrinolysis. *Gastroenterology.* 2001 Jul;121(1):131-9.

[22] Lisman T, Porte RJ. Activation and regulation of hemostasis in acute liver failure and acute pancreatitis. *Semin Thromb Hemost.* 2010 Jun;36(4):437-43.

[23] Lisman T, Porte RJ. Rebalanced hemostasis in patients with liver disease: evidence and clinical consequences. *Blood.* 2010 Aug 12;116(6):878-85.

[24] Lodge JP, Jonas S, Oussoultzoglou E, Malago M, Jayr C, Cherqui D, et al. Recombinant coagulation factor VIIa in major liver resection: a randomized, placebo-controlled, double-blind clinical trial. *Anesthesiology.* 2005 Feb;102(2):269-75.

[25] Longo DL. Harrison's principles of internal medicine. 18th ed. New York: McGraw-Hill; 2012.

[26] Loscalzo J, Vaughan DE. Tissue Plasminogen-Activator Promotes Platelet Disaggregation in Plasma. *J Clin Invest.* 1987 Jun;79(6):1749-55.

[27] Mammen EF. Coagulation defects in liver disease. *Med Clin North Am.* 1994 May;78(3):545-54.

[28] Mammen EF. Coagulopathies of liver disease. *Clin Lab Med.* 1994 Dec;14(4):769-80.

[29] Mannucci PM. Abnormal hemostasis tests and bleeding in chronic liver disease: are they related? No. *J Thromb Haemost.* 2006 Apr;4(4):721-3.

[30] Mannucci PM, Remuzzi G, Pusineri F, Lombardi R, Valsecchi C, Mecca G, et al. Deamino-8-D-arginine vasopressin shortens the bleeding time in uremia. *N Engl J Med*. 1983 Jan 6;308(1):8-12.

[31] Marder VJ, Sherry S. Thrombolytic Therapy - Current Status .1. *New Engl J Med*. 1988 Jun 9;318(23):1512-20.

[32] Munoz SJ, Ballas SK, Moritz MJ, Martinez J, Friedman LS, Jarrell BE, et al. Perioperative management of fulminant and subfulminant hepatic failure with therapeutic plasmapheresis. *Transplant Proc*. 1989 Jun;21(3):3535-6.

[33] Munoz SJ, Stravitz RT, Gabriel DA. Coagulopathy of acute liver failure. *Clin Liver Dis*. 2009 Feb;13(1):95-107.

[34] Nair SC, Dargaud Y, Chitlur M, Srivastava A. Tests of global haemostasis and their applications in bleeding disorders. *Haemophilia*. 2010 Jul;16 Suppl 5:85-92.

[35] O'Connell KA, Wood JJ, Wise RP, Lozier JN, Braun MM. Thromboembolic adverse events after use of recombinant human coagulation factor VIIa. *Jama*. 2006 Jan 18;295(3):293-8.

[36] Pandey S, Vyas GN. Adverse effects of plasma transfusion. *Transfusion*. 2012 May;52 Suppl 1:65S-79S.

[37] Peck-Radosavljevic M, Wichlas M, Zacherl J, Stiegler G, Stohlawetz P, Fuchsjager M, et al. Thrombopoietin induces rapid resolution of thrombocytopenia after orthotopic liver transplantation through increased platelet production. *Blood*. 2000 Feb 1;95(3):795-801.

[38] Pereboom IT, de Boer MT, Haagsma EB, Hendriks HG, Lisman T, Porte RJ. Platelet transfusion during liver transplantation is associated with increased postoperative mortality due to acute lung injury. *Anesth Analg*. 2009 Apr;108(4):1083-91.

[39] Qamar AA, Grace ND, Groszmann RJ, Garcia-Tsao G, Bosch J, Burroughs AK, et al. Incidence, Prevalence, and Clinical Significance of Abnormal Hematologic Indices in Compensated Cirrhosis. *Clin Gastroenterol H*. 2009 Jun;7(6):689-95.

[40] Rake MO, Flute PT, Shilkin KB, Lewis ML, Winch J, Williams R. Early and intensive therapy of intravascular coagulation in acute liver failure. *Lancet*. 1971 Dec 4;2(7736):1215-8.

[41] Reverter JC. Abnormal hemostasis tests and bleeding in chronic liver disease: are they related? Yes. *J Thromb Haemost*. 2006 Apr;4(4):717-20.

[42] Segal JB, Dzik WH. Paucity of studies to support that abnormal coagulation test results predict bleeding in the setting of invasive

procedures: an evidence-based review. *Transfusion.* 2005 Sep;45(9):1413-25.

[43] Senzolo M, Burra P, Cholongitas E, Burroughs AK. New insights into the coagulopathy of liver disease and liver transplantation. *World J Gastroenterol.* 2006 Dec 28;12(48):7725-36.

[44] Singal AK, Kamath PS, Tefferi A. Mesenteric venous thrombosis. *Mayo Clin Proc.* 2013 Mar;88(3):285-94.

[45] Stahel PF, Moore EE, Schreier SL, Flierl MA, Kashuk JL. Transfusion strategies in postinjury coagulopathy. *Curr Opin Anaesthesiol.* 2009 Apr;22(2):289-98.

[46] Stricker RB, Wong D, Shiu DT, Reyes PT, Shuman MA. Activation of Plasminogen by Tissue Plasminogen-Activator on Normal and Thrombasthenic Platelets - Effects on Surface-Proteins and Platelet-Aggregation. *Blood.* 1986 Jul;68(1):275-80.

[47] Swallow RA, Agarwala RA, Dawkins KD, Curzen NP. Thromboelastography: potential bedside tool to assess the effects of antiplatelet therapy? *Platelets.* 2006 Sep;17(6):385-92.

[48] Tripodi A. The coagulopathy of chronic liver disease: is there a causal relationship with bleeding? No. *Eur J Intern Med.* 2010 Apr;21(2):65-9.

[49] Tripodi A, Chantarangkul V, Mannucci PM. The international normalized ratio to prioritize patients for liver transplantation: problems and possible solutions. *J Thromb Haemost.* 2008 Feb;6(2):243-8.

[50] Tripodi A, Mannucci PM. The coagulopathy of chronic liver disease. *N Engl J Med.* 2011 Jul 14;365(2):147-56.

[51] Tripodi A, Primignani M, Chantarangkul V, Clerici M, Dell'Era A, Fabris F, et al. Thrombin generation in patients with cirrhosis: the role of platelets. *Hepatology.* 2006 Aug;44(2):440-5.

[52] Tripodi A, Primignani M, Chantarangkul V, Dell'Era A, Clerici M, de Franchis R, et al. An imbalance of pro- vs anti-coagulation factors in plasma from patients with cirrhosis. *Gastroenterology.* 2009 Dec;137(6):2105-11.

[53] Tripodi A, Salerno F, Chantarangkul V, Clerici M, Cazzaniga M, Primignani M, et al. Evidence of normal thrombin generation in cirrhosis despite abnormal conventional coagulation tests. *Hepatology.* 2005 Mar;41(3):553-8.

[54] Trotter JF. Coagulation abnormalities in patients who have liver disease. *Clin Liver Dis.* 2006 Aug;10(3):665-78, x-xi.

[55] Vassiliadis T, Mpoumponaris A, Vakalopoulou S, Giouleme O, Gkissakis D, Grammatikos N, et al. Spur cells and spur cell anemia in

hospitalized patients with advanced liver disease: Incidence and correlation with disease severity and survival. *Hepatol Res.* 2010 Feb;40(2):161-70.

[56] Violi F, Basili V, Ferro D, Quintarelli C, Alessandri C, Cordova C. Association between high values of D-dimer and Tissue-plasminogen activator activity and first gastrointestinal bleeding in cirrhotic patients. *Thromb Haemostasis.* 1996 Aug;76(2):177-83.

[57] Wu H, Nguyen GC. Liver cirrhosis is associated with venous thromboembolism among hospitalized patients in a nationwide US study. *Clin Gastroenterol Hepatol.* 2010 Sep;8(9):800-5.

[58] Zambruni A, Thalheimer U, Coppell J, Riddell A, Mancuso A, Leandro G, et al. Endogenous heparin-like activity detected by anti-Xa assay in infected cirrhotic and non-cirrhotic patients. *Scand J Gastroenterol.* 2004 Sep;39(9):830-6.

[59] Zeigler ZR, Megaludis A, Fraley DS. Desmopressin (d-DAVP) effects on platelet rheology and von Willebrand factor activities in uremia. *Am J Hematol.* 1992 Feb;39(2):90-5.

In: Disseminated Intravascular Coagulation (DIC)   ISBN: 978-1-62948-323-8
Editor: Balwinder Singh   © 2014 Nova Science Publishers, Inc.

Chapter VIII

Disseminated Intravascular Coagulation in Urological Malignancy

Aydin Pooli MD[1] *and Dharam Kaushik MD*[*2]
[1]Division of Urology, University of Nebraska Medical Center,
Omaha, Nebraska, US
[2] Department of Urology, Mayo Clinic,
Rochester, Minnesota, US

Abstract

Disseminated intravascular coagulopathy (DIC) can impose a significant burden of morbidity to the patients with urologic malignancies. Although there are reports of DIC in different urologic malignancies, it is most commonly seen in prostate cancer (PCa) with an incidence of approximately 13% to 30%. However, only 0.4 to 1.6% of patients with PCa may present with clinical signs and symptoms of DIC. The incidence of DIC is shown to increase with higher Gleason score, stage and presence of metastatic disease. The underlying pathophysiology of DIC in PCa is related to the presence of pro-coagulants capable of

---

* Correspondence: Dr. Dharam Kaushik, MD, Department of Urology, Mayo Clinic, Rochester, Minnesota, 55902, USA; Email: drdkuro@gmail.com.

directly activating factor X, tissue factor expression by malignant cells, secretion of pro-aggregation factors, pro-inflammatory cytokines and direct interaction of malignant cells with red blood cells. In chronic DIC these pathways are more balanced and compensatory mechanisms are able to restore platelets and coagulation factors. The diagnosis of DIC is made by decreased platelet count, increased fibrin related markers including fibrin degradation products, D-dimer, soluble fibrin, decreased fibrinogen, and increased Prothrombin Time (PT). Treatment of DIC should be focused on treating the primary cancer. Supportive therapy involves platelets transfusion, fresh frozen plasma (FFP) or prothrombin complex concentrate for patients with predominantly bleeding features and anticoagulation for patients with features of thrombosis.

Introduction

Disseminated intravascular coagulopathy (DIC) may impose a significant risk and life threatening complications in cancer patients. Urologic malignancies are not an exception in this regard. Although cancer patients may suffer from a variety of coagulate complications including thrombotic thrombocytopenic purpura (TTP), deep venous thrombosis (DVT) and acquired coagulation factor deficiencies, DIC remains the most common coagulopathy in urological cancer patients [1].

Since DIC is caused by abnormal activation of coagulation system through exposure to pro-coagulants, it leads to thrombosis formation and eventually consumption of coagulative factors causing bleeding tendency. Abnormal thrombus formation and consumption coagulopathy is usually a catastrophic event, especially in cancer patients.

Malignancy is the third most common cause of DIC after infection and trauma. Malignancies predispose patients to a variety of hypercoagulable state consisting of DVT, DIC, thrombotic microangiopathy and arterial thrombus. However, the pathogenesis of these hypercoagulable states is multifactorial and involves a complex interplay of cancer type, comorbidities, medications, infection, and surgical approaches. [2, 3]

In this chapter, we will review the epidemiology, pathophysiology, clinical presentation and management of DIC in urological cancer.

Prostate Cancer

Epidemiology

Prostate cancer (PCa) is the most commonly diagnosed cancer in males and historically is reported to be associated with coagulation disorders. [4]Migratory thrombophlebitis, venous thrombosis, non-bacterial endocarditis, arterial thrombosis/emboli and DIC have been reported with PCa. [5-7] DIC can present as an initial manifestation of advanced prostate cancer. Commonly in an undiagnosed PCa patient, it presents by excessive bleeding following prostate biopsy. [8]. Approximately 45% of prostate cancer patients who develop DIC will have Gleason score$\geq$8 and majority of patients will have castration-resistant prostate cancer. [9] The incidence of DIC in prostate cancer is reported to be approximately 25% by Straub in 1971 [10] and more recent studies revealed an incidence in the range of 13 to 30%; however, only 0.4 to 1.6 % patients may present with overt clinical signs and symptoms of DIC. [5, 11] Cancer stage plays an important role in PCa, as the incidence increases in higher stages and in metastatic disease. [12] The serum markers historically used to diagnose DIC have been proposed and studied to detect prostate cancer [4, 13].

Pathophysiology

Coagulation system activation in prostate cancer is multifactorial and complex. Cancer cells may produce a cysteine protease as procoagulant that can directly activate factor X. [14, 15] Other mechanisms may include tissue factor expression by tumor cells, fibrinolysis, pro aggregation factors, pro inflammatory cytokines and direct interaction of malignant cells with red blood cells [3].

Host cells and malignant cells can express tissue factor that forms a complex with factor VII to activate factor X and coagulation eventually. However, expression of tissue factor is tightly controlled and only occurs when there is damage to vascular bed, or exposure to pro-inflammatory cytokines such as tumor necrosis factor and interleukin 1B. Tumor cells on the other hand may express tissue factor uncontrolled and constitutively [3] Malignant prostate cells may also express fibrinolytic factors including urokinase, tissue type plasminogen activator, plasminogen receptors and even plasminogen activator inhibitors. [13, 16, 17] D-dimer and fibrinopeptide A have been used to evaluate the activation of coagulation system. D dimer is a peptide released by cleavage of fibrin which is activated by plasmin. Fibrinopeptide A on the other hand is produced by cleavage of the alpha chain of fibrinogen by thrombin. The incidence of coagulopathy in PCa and its clinical significance was studied by Adamson et al. in a prospective study in which hemostasis activation was assessed by D dimer and Fibrinopeptide A. In their study, D dimer and Fibrinopeptide A were significantly higher in PCa patients compared to BPH patients and both markers were significantly higher in patients with positive bone scans. They reported elevated fibrinopeptide A and D dimer in 40 percent and 24 percent of PCa patients respectively with positive correlation with bone scan status. They calculated a positive predictive value of 91 percent between D-dimer and presence of bone metastasis. They conclude that subclinical DIC is quite common in prostate cancer and D dimer and Fibrinopeptide A may be used as tumor marker in prostate cancer. [4] A more recent study by Shariat et al. demonstrated that Urokinase-type plasminogen activator (uPA) and Urokinase type plasminogen activator receptor (uPAR) levels are significantly higher in patients with prostate cancer compared to their normal controls. The study demonstrated that plasma levels of uPA and uPAR are higher in prostate cancers with metastasis and locally advanced cancer compared to localized tumor. In addition, higher plasma levels of uPA and uPAR were associated with biologically aggressive cancers such as higher Gleason scores, lymph node metastases and seminal vesicle involvement. [13] They concluded that uPA and uPAR are most probably prostatic origin as their levels decreased significantly following radical prostatectomy, therefor uPA and uPAR may be considered as bio markers of aggressive PCa.

Clinical Presentation

Clinical presentation of DIC in prostate cancer may be acute or chronic based on the balance between intravascular coagulation and depletion of coagulation factors and platelets. Acute and uncontrolled activation of thrombotic pathways leads to intra vascular coagulation leading to consumption of coagulation factors as well as platelets, which leads to bleeding tendency. In chronic DIC, on the other hand, coagulopathy is more controlled and compensatory mechanisms restore the coagulation factors and platelets. [5, 19]

Renal Cell Carcinoma

Various types of coagulopathy may be seen in renal cell carcinoma (RCC), majority of which are caused either by lupus anicoagulant (auto immune antibody formation) or due to Stauffer's syndrome. Lupus anticoagulant syndrome (LAS) occasionally occurs in RCC as a paraneoplastic syndrome with increased PTT and higher than normal chances of thromboembolism. [19]

Liver dysfunction in presence of RCC, known as Stauffer syndrome, is also associated with coagulopathy in which increased prothrombin time is not due to tumor infiltration of the liver or depletion of vitamin K dependent coagulation factors but increased fibrin degradation factor complexes suggest compensated intravascular coagulation possibly triggered by tumor cells [20] Autoimmune hemolytic anemia is another paraneoplastic phenomenon secondary to warm and cold auto antibodies observed in RCC. Antibodies to platelets and to C1 esterase inhibitor also may contribute to coagulopathy in RCC. [21]

Since DIC is thought to be secondary to paraneoplastic syndrome in RCC, removing the neoplastic tissue can completely or partially ameliorate the signs and symptoms of DIC. In the meantime regular management of DIC including depleting coagulation factors and anticoagulation should not be overlooked.

Wilms Tumor

Wilms tumor is the most common renal malignancy in childhood which is usually asymptomatic and diagnosed incidentally as a palpable abdominal mass. [22-24]. It may present with abdominal pain, high blood pressure and may be associated with polycythemia, intratumor hemorrhage and acquired von Willebrand disease which makes the patient prone to bleeding diathesis [22-26]

The mechanism for acquired von Willebrand factor deficiency has been proposed to include immunologic activation of VW factor, impaired release from tissue storage sites, proteolysis and absorption by tumor cells. [23, 27, 28]

Miscellaneous Urological Causes of DIC

Literature on DIC in other urological malignancies is scant and mainly consists of case reports. Lee et al. published the first reported case of adrenal cortical malignancy with DIC as a fatal manifestation. They reported a 54-year-old man who was admitted to hospital with back pain, and several bruises on the trunk and extremities who was found to have increased fibrin degradation products, and D dimer as well as a left adrenal mass in abdominal CT scan. Their patient died due to pulmonary thromboembolic event and respiratory distress; post mortem autopsy revealed a left adrenal cystic mass with multiple pulmonary metastatic nodules consistent with pleomorphic adrenal carcinoma. [29] They suggested that although DIC is a rare presentation in adrenal cortical tumors, it should be considered in differential diagnosis. Microangiopathic hemolytic anemia (MAHA) secondary to DIC was reported in a case of malignant pheochromocytoma with bone metastasis by Sakai et al. [30] DIC has also been reported in mesoblastic nephroma in neonates and infants in 2 case reports. In both of these cases, the patients demonstrated good prognosis and favorable outcomes. [31, 32] Vora et al. reported two cases of neonatal neuroblastoma with bleeding tendency due to DIC and concluded that although rare, hemorrhagic events and DIC can be a major manifestation in neuroblastoma. [33] Tumor manipulation during radical cystectomy was suggested to constitute as the triggering factor for DIC for bladder papillary carcinoma by Tauzin-Fin et al. causing thrombotic micro angiopathy. [34]

Diagnosis and Treatment of DIC in Urological Patient

DIC is an important problem in urological malignancies. Acute DIC can be catastrophic in a patient who already has a urologic malignancy therefore, early diagnosis and treatment of DIC is extremely important. In addition diagnosis of subclinical and chronic DIC is important as the management strategy may differ. [35, 37]

Scientific and Standardization Committee of International Society on Thrombosis and Hemostasis (ISTH) has divided the definition of DIC into two sub categories: Overt DIC which is a state of decompensated coagulation system and non-overt DIC where the coagulation system is in compensated state. [38]

Overt DIC is diagnosed by decreased platelet count, increased fibrin related markers including fibrin degradation products, D-dimer, soluble fibrin, decreased fibrinogen, and increased PT. A score of 5 or less in ISTH guidelines indicates non-overt DIC whereas score more than 5 is compatible with overt DIC [38].

Active treatment of underlying disease plays an essential role in treatment of DIC. For example, prostatectomy in clinically localized PCa will eliminate the tumor cells making the patient prone to DIC. However, in metastatic cancers or non-operable patients, excision of the malignant tissues may not be possible. In addition, patients with malignancies may receive chemotherapy, radiation therapy or hormone replacement or ablation therapy which makes patients more likely to develop DIC.

Current recommendations for DIC management include transfusion of platelets in patients with ongoing and active bleeding in case of low platelet count (less than 50000/ml), administration of Fresh Frozen Plasma in cases of prolonged PT/APTT or decreased fibrinogen. In cases that FFP transfusion is not possible, prothrombin complex concentrate may be considered.

In patients with malignancy related DIC and thrombosis predominance therapeutic dose of anticoagulants including low molecular weight heparin (LMWH) or unfractionated heparin (UH) are usually considered. However, LMWH is preferred due to high quality and low risk of heparin induced thrombocytopenia. Prophylactic doses of LMWH or UF must be seriously considered in debilitated, critically ill patients with subclinical or non-hemorrhagic DIC [39, 40]

References

[1]   Bick RL. Disseminated intravascular coagulation: a review of etiology, pathophysiology, diagnosis, and management: guidelines for care. *Clin Appl Thromb Hemost.* 2002 Jan;8(1):1-31.

[2]   Young A, Chapman O, Connor C, Poole C, Rose P, Kakkar AK. Thrombosis and cancer. *Nat Rev Clin Oncol.* 2012 Aug;9(8):437-49.

[3]   Prandoni P, Falanga A, Piccioli A. Cancer and venous thromboembolism. *Lancet Oncol.* 2005 Jun;6(6):401-10.

[4]   Adamson AS, Francis JL, Witherow RO, Snell ME. Coagulopathy in the prostate cancer patient: prevalence and clinical relevance. *Ann R Coll Surg Engl.* 1993 Mar;75(2):100-4.

[5]   de la Fouchardiere C, Flechon A, Droz JP. Coagulopathy in prostate cancer. *Neth J Med.* 2003 Nov;61(11):347-54.

[6]   Smith JA, Jr., Soloway MS, Young MJ. Complications of advanced prostate cancer. *Urology.* 1999 Dec;54(6A Suppl):8-14.

[7]   Sun NC, McAfee WM, Hum GJ, Weiner JM. Hemostatic abnormalities in malignancy, a prospective study of one hundred eight patients. Part I. Coagulation studies. *Am J Clin Pathol.* 1979 Jan;71(1):10-6.

[8]   Al-Otaibi MF, Al-Taweel W, Bin-Saleh S, Herba M, Aprikian AG. Disseminated intravascular coagulation following transrectal ultrasound guided prostate biopsy. *J Urol.* 2004 Jan;171(1):346.

[9]   Hyman DM, Soff GA, Kampel LJ. Disseminated intravascular coagulation with excessive fibrinolysis in prostate cancer: a case series and review of the literature. *Oncology.* 2011;81(2):119-25.

[10]   Straub PW. Chronic intravascular coagulation. Clinical spectrum and diagnostic criteria, with special emphasis on metabolism, distribution and localization of I 131 -fibrinogen. *Acta Med Scand Suppl.* 1971;526:1-95.

[11]   Ruffion A, Manel A, Valignat C, Lopez JG, Perrin-Fayolle O, Perrin P. Successful use of Samarium 153 for emergency treatment of disseminated intravascular coagulation due to metastatic hormone refractory prostate cancer. *J Urol.* 2000 Sep;164(3 Pt 1):782.

[12]   Cabane J, Etarian C, Louvet C, Robert A, Blum L, Wattiaux MJ, et al. [Disseminated intravascular coagulation associated with prostatic cancer]. *Rev Med Interne.* 1995;16(3):219-24.

[13]   Shariat SF, Roehrborn CG, McConnell JD, Park S, Alam N, Wheeler TM, et al. Association of the circulating levels of the urokinase system of plasminogen activation with the presence of prostate cancer and invasion, progression, and metastasis. *J Clin Oncol.* 2007 Feb 1;25(4):349-55.

[14]   Gordon SG, Franks JJ, Lewis B. Cancer procoagulant A: a factor X activating procoagulant from malignant tissue. *Thromb Res.* 1975 Feb;6(2):127-37.

[15]   Gordon SG, Franks JJ, Lewis BJ. Comparison of procoagulant activities in extracts of normal and malignant human tissue. *J Natl Cancer* Inst. 1979 Apr;62(4):773-6.

[16] Hienert G, Kirchheimer JC, Pfluger H, Binder BR. Urokinase-type plasminogen activator as a marker for the formation of distant metastases in prostatic carcinomas. *J Urol.* 1988 Dec;140(6):1466-9.

[17] Kirchheimer J, Koller A, Binder BR. Isolation and characterization of plasminogen activators from hyperplastic and malignant prostate tissue. *Biochim Biophys Acta.* 1984 Feb 14;797(2):256-65.

[18] Peck SD, Reiquam CW. Disseminated intravascular coagulation in cancer patients: supportive evidence. *Cancer.* 1973 May;31(5):1114-9.

[19] Berdjis N, Meier M, Hoeppner F, Behrendt H. [Coagulopathy resulting from lupus anticoagulant antibodies as a paraneoplastic phenomenon in renal cell carcinoma relapse]. *Urologe A.* 2008 Jan;47(1):65-7.

[20] Andrassy K, Gartner H, Siede WH, Ritz E, Riedasch G, Mohring K, et al. Stauffer's syndrome in renal cell carcinoma evidence for intravascular coagulation. *Klin Wochenschr.* 1980 Jan 15;58(2):91-7.

[21] Puthenparambil J, Lechner K, Kornek G. Autoimmune hemolytic anemia as a paraneoplastic phenomenon in solid tumors: A critical analysis of 52 cases reported in the literature. *Wien Klin Wochenschr.* 2010 Apr;122(7-8):229-36.

[22] Angell SK, Pruthi RS, Merguerian PA. Pediatric genitourinary tumors. *Curr Opin Oncol.* 1996 May;8(3):240-6.

[23] Leung RS, Liesner R, Brock P. Coagulopathy as a presenting feature of Wilms tumour. *Eur J Pediatr.* 2004 Jul;163(7):369-73.

[24] Shamberger RC. Pediatric renal tumors. *Semin Surg Oncol.* 1999 Mar;16(2):105-20.

[25] Coppes MJ, Zandvoort SW, Sparling CR, Poon AO, Weitzman S, Blanchette VS. Acquired von Willebrand disease in Wilms' tumor patients. *J Clin Oncol.* 1992 Mar;10(3):422-7.

[26] Jonge Poerink-Stockschlader AB, Dekker I, Risseeuw-Appel IM, Hahlen K. Acquired Von Willebrand disease in children with a Wilms' tumor. *Med Pediatr Oncol.* 1996 Apr;26(4):238-43.

[27] Handin RI, Martin V, Moloney WC. Antibody-induced von Willebrand's disease: a newly defined inhibitor syndrome. *Blood.* 1976 Sep;48(3):393-405.

[28] Stableforth P, Tamagnini GL, Dormandy KM. Acquired von Willebrand syndrome with inhibitors both to factor VIII clotting activity and ristocetin-induced platelet aggregation. *Br J Haematol.* 1976 Aug;33(4):565-73.

[29] Lee KW, Chon SB, Kim DY, Yun T, Yoon SS, Park S, et al. Adrenal cortical carcinoma initially presented with overwhelming disseminated intravascular coagulation. *Ann Hematol.* 2003 Sep;82(9):596-8.

[30] Sakai C, Takagi T, Oguro M, Wakatsuki S, Kuwahara T. Malignant pheochromocytoma accompanied by microangiopathic hemolytic anemia: a case report. *Jpn J Clin Oncol.* 1994 Jun;24(3):171-4.

[31] Sailer R, Voigt HJ, Scharf J, Hummer HP, Schmitzer E, Beck JD. [Disseminated intravascular coagulation caused by prenatal hemorrhage into a congenital mesoblastic nephroma. Case report]. *Klin Padiatr.* 1993 May-Jun;205(3):176-9.

[32] Zach TL, Cifuentes RF, Strom RL. Congenital mesoblastic nephroma, hemorrhagic shock, and disseminated intravascular coagulation in a newborn infant. *Am J Perinatol.* 1991 May;8(3):203-5.

[33] Vora D, Slovis TL, Boal DK. Hemoperitoneum and disseminated intravascular coagulation in two neonates with congenital bilateral neuroblastoma. *Pediatr Radiol.* 2000 Jun;30(6):394-7.

[34] Tauzin-Fin P, Sesay M, Ryman A, Ballanger P, Combe C. Postoperative thrombotic microangiopathy following radical cystectomy for bladder cancer. *Anaesth Intensive Care.* 2006 Oct;34(5):672-5.

[35] Kaneko T, Wada H. Diagnostic criteria and laboratory tests for disseminated intravascular coagulation. *J Clin Exp Hematop.* 2011;51(2):67-76.

[36] Saito H, Maruyama I, Shimazaki S, Yamamoto Y, Aikawa N, Ohno R, et al. Efficacy and safety of recombinant human soluble thrombomodulin (ART-123) in disseminated intravascular coagulation: results of a phase III, randomized, double-blind clinical trial. *J Thromb Haemost.* 2007 Jan;5(1):31-41.

[37] Warren BL, Eid A, Singer P, Pillay SS, Carl P, Novak I, et al. Caring for the critically ill patient. High-dose antithrombin III in severe sepsis: a randomized controlled trial. *JAMA.* 2001 Oct 17;286(15):1869-78.

[38] Taylor FB, Jr., Toh CH, Hoots WK, Wada H, Levi M. Towards definition, clinical and laboratory criteria, and a scoring system for disseminated intravascular coagulation. *Thromb Haemost.* 2001 Nov;86(5):1327-30.

[39] Kawasugi K, Wada H, Hatada T, Okamoto K, Uchiyama T, Kushimoto S, et al. Prospective evaluation of hemostatic abnormalities in overt DIC due to various underlying diseases. *Thromb Res.* 2011 Aug;128(2):186-90.

[40] Wada H, Thachil J, Di Nisio M, Mathew P, Kurosawa S, Gando S, et al. Guidance for diagnosis and treatment of DIC from harmonization of the recommendations from three guidelines. *J Thromb Haemost.* 2013 Feb 4.

In: Disseminated Intravascular Coagulation (DIC)   ISBN: 978-1-62948-323-8
Editor: Balwinder Singh   © 2014 Nova Science Publishers, Inc.

Chapter IX

Chronic Disseminated Intravascular Coagulation (DIC) in Solid Tumors: When, Whom and How to Treat?

Felice Vito Vitale, MD, Giovanna Antonelli, MD,*
Rosalba Rossello, MD and Francesco Ferraù, MD
Department of Oncology, Division of Medical Oncology,
San Vincenzo Hospital, Taormina, Italy

Abstract

Most cancer patients suffering from solid tumors are found to have markers of coagulation activation and/or fibrinolysis in their blood samples. This prothrombotic state exists virtually in all patients, being detectable in about 50% of patients with localized tumours and in more than 90% with metastatic disease. So that these patients are diagnosed with subclinical chronic disseminated intravascular coagulation (DIC). Progression to decompensated chronic DIC can occur during the clinical

---

* Correspondence concerning this article should be addressed to Felice Vito Vitale Department of Oncology, Division of Medical Oncology, San Vincenzo Hospital , Contrada Sirina, 98039, Taormina, Italy. f.vitale@videobank.it.

course of malignant diseases. Decompensation of such a chronic DIC can lead to a low intensity decompensated DIC (LIDDIC) or can progress to overt acute and diffuse DIC finally resulting in diffuse haemorrhage and/or thrombosis. Also, chronic DIC may trigger thromboembolic disease. The authors aim to focus on emerging issues and often unanswered questions about when, whom and how to treat chronic DIC.

Keywords: Chronic disseminated intravascular coagulation; solid tumors; decompensated DIC

1. Introduction and Pathophysiology

Abnormal haemostasis is a functional property of cancer. A significant number of cancer patients manifests laboratory evidence of hypercoagulable state and some of them develop thromboembolic complications. Cancer cells have been reported to have biologic properties favouring their interaction with blood coagulation pathways. Tumor cells activate the haemostasis procoagulant pathways directly via procoagulants compounds such as the tissue factor (TF) or cancer procoagulant (CP), and/or indirectly by secreting tumor necrosis factor alpha (TNFα) and interleukin-1 beta (IL-1β), thus upregulating TF expression on endothelial vascular cells and on monocytes [1-3]. Furthermore even fibrinolitic cascade is usually significantly activated in cancer diseases [4].

Different clinical complications may correlate with cancer associated thrombophilic state during the life of cancer patients suffering from solid cancer. Although venous thromboembolism is more frequently observed, even disseminated intravascular coagulation has relevant place in the context of cancer hypercoagulability related complications [5].

2. Definition

The so called chronic DIC is a well known cancer related hypercoagulable state. It is a common consumption coagulopathy characterized by a ceaseless production and removal of fibrin network sometime overflowing into progressive exhaustion of coagulation factors and platelets [2, 6, 7]. Drop in platelets count, prothrombin time (PT) and activated partial thromboplastin time (aPTT) prolongation often along with hypofibrinogenemia, result in a clinical and/or laboratory clear evidence of DIC (overt DIC). The clinical and/or laboratory course of overt DIC might vary from an indolent trend (mild DIC) to a catastrophic thrombocytopenia and bleeding (acute DIC) [8].

For practical use, in order to maintain homogenous definitions in an ever-growing body of literature evidence, the clinical picture known as "low intensity decompensated DIC" could superimpose to the term "mild-DIC" but should be distinguished from "chronic-DIC". While the diagnosis of overt acute DIC may be relatively simple, in front of evident clinical and laboratory pictures and defined guidelines, the diagnosis of low intensity decompensated DIC is often difficult because of lack of consensus as to the appropriate definition and clinical and laboratory criteria for diagnosis. This disorder of blood coagulation is reflected in laboratory findings such as only borderline-low platelets count or their slow progressive drop, elevation in plasma level of fibrinogen degradation products (FDP) and D-dimer, normal or moderately deranged level of other coagulation parameters such as prothrombin time (PT), activated partial thromboplastin time (aPTT), fibrinogen and antithrombin III concentration [7, 9, 10]. Nonetheless, some authors choose the terms non-overt DIC or pre-DIC state when facing an indolent consumption coagulopathy but, in this case, the use of the above terms could be considered questionable [11].

DIC in cancer has, in general, a less dramatic course than when occurring in sepsis and trauma [7]. For this reasons three types of DIC related to cancer patients should be distinguished: early (non-overt) compensated DIC, low intensity decompensated DIC or "mild" DIC and acute DIC. Both of the latter two coagulopathies can be classified as overt DIC. Lots of updated laboratory tests, namely haemostatic molecular markers such as antithrombin (AT), thrombomodulin (TM), thrombin-antithrombin complex (TAT), plasmin-plasmin inhibitor complex (PPIC), soluble fibrin (SF), prothrombin fragments 1+2 (F1+2), whose expression levels are significantly different in accordance with variable stages and intensity of consumption coagulopathy, are going to be included in diagnostic algorithms able to better define the different clotting derangements [9, 12-14]. With the relevant expanding field of new therapeutic options in medical oncology, with an overwhelming role to be assumed by targeted therapies, the knowledge of the sometimes subtle differentiation of these clinical conditions must become a part of Medical Oncologist's education. Clinicians should be alert to the occurrence of such clotting disorders and should be confident with their diagnosis and management.

3. Diagnostic Criteria

The diagnostic criteria with operative purpose now available for definition of DIC suffer of two methodological weakness: first, the pathophysiological mechanisms and the clinical pictures are substantially conditioned by the underlying disease, theoretically requiring a dedicated DIC score for specific disease, while the currently used criteria encompasse common features of different types of DIC; second, these criteria are actually decision tools for starting the treatment of DIC, rather than criteria for diagnosing it.

This conceptual framework descends from the evolution in the clinical diagnostic and therapeutical approach to DIC. While the picture of overt acute DIC is well-known and easy-to-diagnose on clinical ground since almost three decades, most recently clinicians tend to utilize laboratory criteria to easier intercept the DIC onset, well before clinical appearance. In this way, they are able to identify the coagulopathy in its earliest or indolent stages as "pre-DIC" or "low intensity decompensated DIC", and to counteract these ones with potentially more efficacious therapeutical measures.

Early therapeutical approach to this non overt-DIC is of outmost importance, since it is demonstrated that its treatment substantially could reduce the mortality at least in patients suffering from sepsis related consumption coagulopathy; conversely, the rate of DIC remission with therapy is inversely related to the DIC score at the beginning of treatment [9, 15, 16,]. Wada et al. recently analyzed in depth three valuable guidelines concerning DIC diagnosis and treatment issued from the British Committee for Standards in Haematology (BCSH), the Japanese Society of Thrombosis and Hemostasis (JSTH), and the Italian Society for Thrombosis and Haemostasis (SISET). All of the mentioned guidelines represent an useful tool for the diagnosis of DIC due to infective and non-infective etiologies [10]. However, as concerns cancer related non acutely decompensated DIC, namely LIDDIC or "mild" DIC, those guidelines do not provide oncologists with sufficiently appropriate diagnostic criteria.

In this regard it is just to remember the potential confounding role of chemotherapy and radiotherapy in contributing to the occurrence of thrombocytopenia. So, the oncologist's clinical diagnostic judgement still maintains a pivotal role when approaching a suspected disseminated coagulation especially in patients suffering from the indolent one.

4. Therapeutic Strategies

Therapy of DIC usually focuses on treating and hopefully reversing the underlying disease in conjunction with supportive treatment, mainly based on frozen fresh plasma (FFP) and platelets infusion, to restore the coagulation factors consumption [17-20]. In cancer patients a subclinical or gradual slow decompensation of coagulation parameters is often recorded. In general, therapeutic approaches should vary according to different clinical and laboratory scenarios [10, 21].

4.1. Chronic Not Decompensated DIC

There is not mandatory indication for treating chronic not decompensated DIC in solid tumors. However it is well known that about 5-15% of cancer patients encounter overt thromboembolic complications and no less than 50% of them are found suffering from venous thromboembolic disease at autopsy [22-25]. Furthermore, the mere observation of certain consumption coagulopathy related laboratory abnormalities, such as markers of coagulation activation fibrinopeptide A (FPA), prothrombin activation fragments 1+2 (F 1+2), thrombin antithrombin complexes or D-Dimers, might not need any therapeutic intervention [23, 26, 27]. So, the single patient's risk of thromboembolic event occurrence should drive the decision whether to start an anticoagulant prophylaxis or not.

Thus, a combination of factors such as clinical parameters and hemostatic biomarkers might be considered as predictive of thromboembolic complications for patients suffering from cancer and even more from not decompensated chronic DIC. Some authors have recently suggested some criteria for scouting cancer patients at high risk for hypercoagulability related complication such as thromboembolism or acute DIC [28-30].

In accordance with the study of Khorana et al., cancer patients undergoing chemotherapy are defined at risk when encountering a cumulative risk score $\geq$ 3 (platelet and white blood cell count, cancer histology, hemoglobin level, administration of erythropoiesis-stimulating agents (ESAs) along with body mass index are the criteria established for assessing the single patient's risk) [30]. Other authors as Barni et al., in addition, underlined the role of certain chemotherapy drugs in enhancing the risk of thromboembolism. [i.e., platinum based compounds and gemcitabine] [31]. Also, some studies suggest even a possible role for significant D-dimer and Prothrombin Fragment 1-2 elevation in predicting high risk of thromboembolic event [6, 32].

Low molecular weight heparin administration could be offered to high risk patient population for reducing the incidence of thrombosis [31]. As regards the condition called as pre-DIC (non overt DIC), often preceding overt decompensated DIC, there are no consistent data to estimate effectiveness of its early treatment in cancer patients although several hemostatic molecular markers have been identified [7, 9, 33].

4.2. Chronic Decompensated DIC

Decompensated DIC in solid tumors most often occur in advanced metastatic disease [34]. Notably, decompensation of Chronic DIC manifests itself mainly in two joints: or as classic overt and acute DIC or as "low intensity decompensated" DIC (also called mild DIC).

The first one requires a prompt treatment. It is characterized by fast derangement of Coagulation parameter, potentially leading to life-threatening bleeding and multi-organ failure. The second one consists in a mild decompensation of chronically activated blood coagulation. It is not unusual during cancer patients clinical course, most of the time has not a dramatic course without requiring therapeutic intervention [7, 35-37]. So, this low intensity decompensated chronic DIC has usually an indolent clinical course, its treatment should not be considered mandatory and some considerations have to cooperate when deciding which type of approach could be the best for this coagulopathy.

Some rules, such as treatment of the underlying condition and blood component therapy as necessary, apply generally to all types of decompensated DIC. At present, guidelines issued by international scientific societies offer useful criteria, based on laboratory and clinical features, for choosing the right therapeutic strategy in treating DIC worsening towards bleeding or severe thrombocytopenia. A blood component therapy based on transfusion of platelets is strongly recommended in DIC patients with "active bleeding and a platelet count of $<50 \times 10^9$/l or in those ones with a high risk of bleeding and a platelet count of $<20 \times 10^9$/l".

Furthermore, FFP administration has to be considered in bleeding patients with prolonged prothrombin time or activated partial thromboplastin time and in those ones at high risk of bleeding" [10, 20]. Moreover, factor concentrates can be administered in the event of FFP administration ineffectiveness while the role of heparin or antithrombin administration in treating DIC is still controversial [10, 20]. Despite the above mentioned guidelines are significantly helpful, the cancer patients suffering from decompensated DIC have different specificities over non-cancer patients that influence the physicians' decision. All of the chemotherapeutic agents and a number of recent biologic antineoplastic or cancer targeted therapeutic agents have the potential to produce thrombocytopenia [38-40]. Of course, the higher risk of rapidly enhancing an ongoing thrombocytopenia is related to traditional chemotherapeutic drugs administration [37, 41]. In this latter case, referring to solid tumors treatment, oncologists may get concerned that the chemotherapy expected benefit in order to stop consumption coagulopathy might be nullified [42]. Therefore, after balancing risks and benefits, it is needed to carefully identify the patients eligible for both antineoplastic therapy and consumption coagulopathy directed treatments.

So, it is worth making some considerations from which moving to practical application in daily clinical practice to better deal with such challenging dilemmas. In particular regard to low intensity decompensated DIC, both patient and tumor-related factors influence physicians' decisions on therapeutic measures. With respect to patient characteristics, life expectancy, performance status and patient fitness for traditional chemotherapy or more generally antineoplastic therapies are relevant data elements that need to be taken into considerations. Also, cancer stage, cancer chemosensitivity profile (in accordance with cancer histotype), previous antineoplastic treatments and their outcome could be the other valuable criteria leading to a more or less intensive management of the low intensity decompensated consumption coagulopathy. On the basis of the above considerations, unpretreated cancer patients fitness for antineoplastic therapies and suffering from tumors significantly responsive to any available antineoplastic treatment should be offered the most significant efforts to overcome or at least improve the consumption coagulopathy. On the contrary, for late stage and/or heavily pretreated cancer patients and those ones suffering from cancer refractory to current antineoplastic agents, watchful waiting may be an appropriate management approach. Possible treatment options have to be centered always on the current guidelines recommendations eventually adapted for the specificity of cancer related therapy. It has to be underlined that cancer patients suffering from LIDDIC eligible for chemotherapy are perceived as potentially at risk for worsening thrombocytopenia and subsequent bleeding. So, in accordance with current guidelines, these kind of patients could be administered fresh frozen plasma [10,20]. Still, administration of low-dose heparin might be considered [10, 20]. Both types of heparin, unfractionated (UFH) or low molecular weight heparin (LMWH), are administrable. Notably, UFH continuous endovenous infusion seems to be safer than LMWH when the risk of bleeding is high thanks to its short half-life and reversibility [20]. The role of other therapeutic strategies, as protein C concentrate, thrombomodulin or inhibitors of tissue factor, remains to be better established in further clinical trials [10]. Of course, concurrently with the above supportive treatment, only a chemotherapy regimen characterized by effectiveness and low myelotoxicity should be used [42].

Conclusion

Chronic DIC is almost constitutively activated in advanced tumors, especially the mucinous ones [43]. The diagnostic algorithm of chronic DIC or acutely decompensated DIC is adequately defined by current guidelines and recommendations which are applicable regardless of DIC etiology. On the contrary when oncologists come across a DIC having an indolent course such as LIDDIC some diagnostic difficulties can appear as cancer patients often undergo many conditions favouring thrombocytopenia. In this case, a clinical judgement also based on the single patient's therapeutic anamnesis and on the knowledge of the metastatic sites has a fundamental role in differential diagnosis. It is really conceivable that only a minority of cancer patients suffering from low Intensity decompensated DIC has a cancer disease potentially responsive to antineoplastic treatment. If so, administration of FFP and/or low dose of UFH and/or LMWH could be taken into account in the attempt of increase platelet count and make antineoplastic drugs administration safer. Unfortunately, most of these patients have a coexisting irreversible disease. Their underlying cancer is usually chemorefractory and already extensively treated. In this case supportive treatment as necessary could be the best choice.

References

[1]   Donati, M.B., Lorenzet, R., (2003). Coagulation factors and tumor cell biology: the role of tissue factor. *Pathophysiol. Haemost. Thromb.* 33 Suppl 1:22-5.

[2]   Falanga, A., (2001). Tumor cell prothrombotic properties. *Hemost.* 31 (1):1-4.

[3]   Falanga, A., Panova-Noeva, M., Russo, L., (2009). Procoagulant mechanisms in tumour cells. *Best Pract. Res. Clin. Haematol.* 22(1):49-60.

[4]   Schmitt, M., Magdolen, V., Mengele, K., Reuning, U., Foekens, J., Diamandis, E. P., Harbeck, N., (2005). Fibrinolytics, enzyme inhibitors, and cancer survival. *Haematol. Rep.* 1(9):28- 33.

[5]   Gupta, P. K., Charan, V. D., Kumar, H., (2005). Cancer Related Thrombophilia : Clinical Importance and Management Strategies. *J. Assoc. Physicians India.* 53:877-82.

[6]   Ay, C., Dunkler, D., Pirker, R., Thaler, J., Quehenberger, P., Wagner, O., Zielinski, C., Pabinger, I., (2012). High D-dimer levels are associated with poor prognosis in cancer patients. *Haematologica.* 97(8):1158-64.

[7]   Levi, M., (2005). Disseminated intravascular coagulation: What's new? *Crit. Care Clin.* 21(3): 449-67.

[8]   Thachil, J., Toh, C.H., (2012). Current concepts in the management of disseminated intravascular coagulation. *Thromb. Res.* 129 Suppl 1:S54-9.

[9]   Wada, H., Hatada, T., Okamoto, K., Uchiyama, T., Kawasugi, K., Mayumi, T., Gando, S., Kushimoto, S., Seki, Y., Madoiwa, S., Okamura, T., Toh, C.H., (2010). Japanese Society of Thrombosis Hemostasis/DIC subcommittee. Modified non-overt DIC diagnostic criteria predict the early phase of overt-DIC. *Am. J. Hematol.* 85(9):691-4.

[10]   Wada, H., Thachil, J., Di Nisio, M., Mathew, P., Kurosawa, S., Gando S., Kim H.K., Nielsen J. D., Dempfle, C. E., Levi, M., Toh, C. H., (2013). The Scientific Standardization Committee on DIC of the International Society on Thrombosis Haemostasis. Guidance for diagnosis and treatment of DIC from harmonization of the recommendations from three guidelines. *J. Thromb. Haemost.* 'Accepted Article', doi: 10.1111/jth.12155.

[11]   Lee, J.H., Song, J., (2010). Diagnosis of non-overt disseminated intravascular coagulation made according to the International Society on Thrombosis and Hemostasis criteria with some modifications. *Korean J. Hematol.* 45(4):260-3.

[12]   Kushimoto, S., Wada, H., Kawasugi, K., Okamoto, K., Uchiyama, T., Seki, Y., Hatada, T., Imai, H., Nobori, T., (2012). Japanese Society of

Thrombosis hemostasis/DIC subcommittee. Increased ratio of soluble fibrin formation/thrombin generation in patient with DIC. *Clin. Appl. Thromb. Hemost.* 18(6):628-32.

[13] Bakhshi, S., Arya, L.S., (2003). Diagnosis and treatment of disseminated intravascular coagulation. *Indian Pediatrics.* 40:721-730.

[14] Lin, S.M., Wang, Y.M., Lin, H.C., Lee, K.Y., Huang, C.D., Liu, C.Y., Wang, C.H., Kuo, H.P., (2008). Serum thrombomodulin level relates to the clinical course of disseminated intravascular coagulation, multiorgan dysfunction syndrome, and mortality in patients with sepsis. *Crit. Care. Med.* 36(3):683-9.

[15] Levi, M., (2005). Prevention of disseminated intravascular coagulation in cancer. *Hematologica reports.* 1(9):52-53.

[16] Wada, H., Wakita, Y., Nakase, T., Shimura, M., Hiyoyama, K., Nagaya, S., Mori, Y., Shiku, H., (1995). Outcome of disseminated intravascular coagulation in relation to the score when treatment was begun. *Thromb. Haemost.*74:848–852.

[17] Wheeler, A., Rubenstein, E. B., (1994). Current management of disseminated intravascular Coagulation. *Oncology (Williston Park).* 8(9):69-73; discussion 73-6 , 79.

[18] Levi, M., de Jonge, E., ten Cate, H., (2000). Disseminated intravascular coagulation. *Ned. Tijdschr. Geneeskd.* 144(10):470-5.

[19] Levi, M., de Jonge, E., (2000). Current management of disseminated intravascular coagulation. *Hosp Pract (Minneap).* 35(8):59-66 ; (quiz 92).

[20] Levi, M., Toh, C.H., Thachil, J., Watson, H.G., (2009).. Guidelines for the diagnosis and management of disseminated intravascular coagulation. British Committee for Standards in Haematology. *Br. J. Haematol.*145(1):24-33.

[21] Levi, M., (2003). Therapeutic options in patients with DIC and cancer. *Pathophysiol. Haemost. Thromb.* 33 Suppl 1:46-7.

[22] Green, K.B., Silverstein, R.L., (1996). Hypercoagulability in cancer. *Hematol. Oncol. Clin. North. Am.*10: 499–530.

[23] Gouin-Thibault, I., Achkar, A., Samama, M.M., (2001). The thrombophilic state in cancer. *Acta Haematol.* 106:33–42.

[24] Peuscher, F.W., (1981). Thrombosis and bleeding in cancer patients. *Neth. J. Med.* 24: 23–35.

[25] Thompson, C.M., Rodgers, R.L., (1952). Analysis of the autopsy records of 157 cases of carcinoma of the pancreas with particular reference to the incidence of thromboembolism. *Am. J. Med. Sci.* 223:469–476.

[26] Luzzatto, G., Schafer, A.I., (1990). The prethrombotic state in cancer. *Semin Oncol.* 17:147-59.

[27] Bick, R.L., (1992). Coagulation abnormalities in malignancy. *Semin. Thromb. Haemost.* 18:353-372.

[28] Connolly, G.C., Khorana, A.A., (2010). Emerging risk stratification approaches to cancer associated thrombosis: risk factors, biomarkers and risk score. *Thromb. Res.* 125 Suppl 2: S1-7.

[29] Ay, C., Pabinger, I. (2012). Predictive potential of haemostatic biomarkers for venous thromboembolism in cancer patients. *Thromb. Res.* 129 Suppl 1:S6-9.

[30] Khorana, A.A., (2012). Risk assessment for cancer-associated thrombosis: what is the best approach? *Thromb. Res.* 129 Suppl 1:S10-5.

[31] Barni, S., Labianca, R., Agnelli, G., Bonizzoni, E., Verso, M., Mandalà, M., Brighenti, M., Petrelli, F., Bianchini, C., Perrone, T., Gasparini, G., (2011). Chemotherapy-associated thromboembolic risk in cancer outpatients and effect of nadroparin thromboprophylaxis: results of a retrospective analysis of the PROTECHT study. *J. Transl. Med.* 20;9:179.

[32] Ay, C., Vormittag, R., Dunkler, D., Simanek, R., Chiriac, A.L., Drach, J., Quehenberger, P., Wagner, O., Zielinski, C., Pabinger, I., (2009). D-dimer and prothrombin fragment 1 + 2 predict venous thromboembolism in patients with cancer: results from the Vienna Cancer and Thrombosis Study. *J. Clin. Oncol.* 27(25):4124-9.

[33] Lee, J.H., Song, J., (2010). Diagnosis of non-overt disseminated intravascular coagulation made according to the International Society on Thrombosis and Hemostasis criteria with some modifications. *Korean J. Hematol.* 45(4):260-3.

[34] Sallah, S., Wan, J.Y., Nguyen, N.P., Hanrahan, L. R., Sigounas, G., (2001). Disseminated intravascular coagulation in solid tumors: clinical and pathologic study. *Thromb. Haemost.* 86(3):828-33.

[35] Francis, J.L., Biggerstaff, J., Amirkhosravi , A., (1998). Hemostasis and malignancy. *Semin. Thromb. Hemost.* 24(2):93-109.

[36] Levi, M., (2001). Cancer and DIC. *Haemost.* 31(suppl. 1):47-48.

[37] Kitchens, C.S., (2009). Thrombocytopenia and thrombosis in disseminated intravascular coagulation (DIC). Hematology *Am Soc Hematol.* Educ. Program. 240-6.

[38] Zeuner, A., Signore, M., Martinetti, D., Bartucci, M., Peschle, C., De Maria, R., (2007). Chemotherapy-induced thrombocytopenia derives

from the selective death of megakaryocyte progenitors and can be rescued by stem cell factor. *Cancer. Res.* 67:4767-4773.

[39] Segota, E., Bukowski, R.M., (2004). The promise of targeted therapy: Cancer drugs become more specific. *Cleve. Clin. J. Med.* 71(7):551-60.

[40] Di Lorenzo, G., Porta, C., Bellmunt, J., Sternberg, C., Kirkali, Z., Staehler, M., Joniau, S., Montorsi, F., Buonerba, C., (2011). Toxicities of targeted therapy and their management in Kidney Cancer. *Eur. Urol.* 59(4):526-40.

[41] Hayashi, S., Ogino, H., Ogata, K., Yagawa, K., (1992). Hypercoagulopathy induced by chemotherapy in a patient with lung cancer. A possible role for a factor with thrombosis-inducing activity (TIA). *Chest.* 101(1):277-8.

[42] Lin, P.H., Lu, Y.S., Lin, C.H., Chang, D.Y., Huang, C.S., Cheng, A.L., Yeh, K.H., (2010). Vinorelbine plus 24-hour infusion of high-dose 5-fluorouracil and leucovorin as effective palliative chemotherapy for breast cancer patients with acute disseminated intravascular coagulation. *Anticancer Res.* 30(7):3087-91.

[43] Varki, A., (2007). Trousseau's syndrome: multiple definitions and multiple mechanisms. *Blood.* 110(6): 1723-9.

In: Disseminated Intravascular Coagulation (DIC)   ISBN: 978-1-62948-323-8
Editor: Balwinder Singh   © 2014 Nova Science Publishers, Inc.

Chapter X

Treatment Options for Disseminated Intravascular Coagulation

Vaibhav Wadhwa MD[*,1] and *Kriti Kalra MD*[2]
[1]Pushpanjali Crosslay Hospital, New Delhi, India
[2]Gundersen Health System, La Crosse, WI, US

Abstract

Disseminated Intravascular Coagulation (DIC) is a life threatening complication that occurs in a wide variety of clinical conditions. DIC predisposes the patients for bleeding, organ failure, shock & thromboembolism and hence has a higher morbidity and mortality. Therefore prevention, early detection and prompt treatment of DIC can increase the chances of patient survival by manifolds. There is a lot of confusion and apprehension that surrounds the management of DIC. The saying 'one size doesn't fit all' stands true in case of DIC. The unpredictable course of the disease process makes it important for the physician to understand that following standard protocol may not give the desired results in all cases. The clinical picture of the patient usually gets

---

[*] Corresponding Author address: Email: vaibhav.manu@gmail.com Dr. Vaibhav Wadhwa, Pushpanjali Crosslay Hospital, New Delhi, India.

precedence over laboratory picture or set guidelines to determine treatment.

Keywords: DIC, treatment, management, coagulation, thrombomodulin

Introduction

Disseminated Intravascular Coagulation (DIC) in easy terms can be defined as coagulation system 'run amok'. DIC is characterized by the widespread activation of coagulation, which results in the intravascular formation of fibrin and ultimately thrombotic occlusion of small and midsize vessels [1]. This in turn leads to inadequate blood supply to organs and ultimately triggering organ failure. In addition, degradation of coagulation proteins occurs along with the widespread activation of the coagulation cascade, which may also result in severe bleeding[1-3].

The management of DIC focuses on three main aspects:

a) Early detection of the etiological factor and its vigorous treatment,
b) Blood products to support the deranged coagulation, and
c) Adequate support to the vital and failing organs.

Treatment Options

General Principles

The management of DIC is an uphill task. The removal of the triggering factor prevents the ongoing pathological process from causing more damage. Whether it is treating sepsis, evacuation of retained products from uterus or managing any other etiological factor causing DIC, this intervention plays a vital role in patient prognosis. While you are getting overwhelmed treating DIC, do NOT forget to support the vital organs i.e., circulation, respiration, renal, liver functions because it is not DIC per se that proves fatal, it is the failed vital organ function that kills a patient. Once the patient has been stabilized, the treatment for DIC should be individualized according to the patient's condition and the etiological factors involved.

Blood Products

The patients with bleeding manifestations have to be supported by blood product administration that includes Platelets, Fresh frozen plasma and Fibrinogen (cryoprecipitate or fibrinogen concentrates)[2].

The clinical condition of the patient is a more important factor in deciding treatment options than the laboratory picture. In patients who are actively bleeding it is advisable to start platelet transfusion at a platelet count below 50 X 10^9/L and below 20 X 10^9/L in patients who are at a high risk for bleeding or awaiting an invasive procedure [4-7]. Instead of a low count, platelet dysfunction could also be the cause for bleeding in DIC and therefore, platelet transfusion can be considered in such patients despite a high platelet count [8].

Fresh Frozen Plasma (FFP) could be given in bleeding patients with a prolonged PT/aPTT (>1.5 times normal) or a decreased fibrinogen level (<1.5g/dL). The recommended dosage is15-20 ml/kg and proper care should be taken not to overload the patient. Consider the same for patients who are not bleeding but need an invasive procedure [4-7].

Cryoprecipitate or Fibrinogen concentrates may be administered to actively bleeding patients who have persistent low fibrinogen levels despite of administration of FFP (<1.5g/dl) [7]. A dose of 3g can raise the plasma fibrinogen level approximately by 1g/L. This can be given as four units of FFP, two cryoprecipitate pools (10 donor units) or as 3g of a fibrinogen concentrate [2]. Prothrombin complex concentrates (PCC) can be considered as an alternative to FFP transfusion in actively bleeding patients if the latter is not possible [7]. Continous monitoring of the patient's coagulation status by repeating platelet count and coagulation profile after component therapy is also an important aspect in management. The initial picture may show a decreased platelet count/coagulation factors/fibrinogen due to continuous thrombin generation [9, 10]. Therefore, a series of lab tests may give a better picture of the patient's coagulation profile rather than a single test.

Vitamin K deficiency should always be ruled out as a cause of prolonged PT before declaring it as DIC.

Specific Drug Therapies

Heparin

There are very specific indications for the use of Heparin in the treatment of DIC. It is mainly recommended for thrombosis predominant DIC. It has proven efficacy in conditions like Purpura fulminans with a significant reduction in mortality from 90% to 18% [11]. Also, heparin plays an important role in DIC related to intrauterine fetal death and hypofibrinogenoma prior to induction of labor, excessive bleeding associated with giant aneurysms and aortic aneurysms (prior to resection) [12]. Of late, Low Molecular Weight Heparin (LMWH) is being preferred over Unfractionated Heparin (UH) as it has a predictable pharmacokinetic profile and a much less risk of bleeding. Dalteparin, a type of LMWH, has already been approved for use in Japan after a multicenter trial showed significant advantages over UH [13]. Prophylaxis with UH or LMWH should be started in critically ill and non-bleeding patients as they are at a high risk for developing venous thromboembolism [2, 14-16]. UH may also be considered in patients with very high risk of bleeding due to its short duration of action and easy reversibility.

Since there is a decrease in antithrombin (AT) in DIC, it is important to make sure that level of AT in the patient is normal or near normal (80-100%) before heparin is used as the anticoagulant action of heparin depends on it's ability to form a complex with AT which then neutralizes the procoagulants [17].

The usual intravenous bolus of UH should be avoided to minimize the bleeding risk [18]. One may use UH in DIC with a weight-adjusted dose of 10μ/kg/h IV, aiming for an aPTT ratio of 1.5-2.5 times the control. Once heparin begins to show its effect, replacement therapy with fresh frozen plasma or cryoprecipitate should be done [2, 7].

Antithrombin

Antithrombin is a major natural anticoagulant which acts by inhibiting thrombin in a 1:1 fashion and leads to thrombin–antithrombin complex (TAT) complex formation with subsequent elimination 19]. The reduction in antithrombin occurs in the early phase of DIC, as there is an excessive generation of thrombin [20]. The level of AT is a strong predictor of mortality especially in cases like sepsis, trauma and major surgery with or without DIC [21, 22]. In these conditions, low levels of AT have been correlated with a poor outcome due to the development of multiple organ failure. Some animal studies have demonstrated that AT can promote the endothelial production of prostacyclin and may therefore have anti-inflammatory actions, hence explaining high efficacy in cases of sepsis. The first randomized controlled trial (RCT) of AT treatment in DIC showed significant reduction in mortality with shorter duration of symptoms and rapid normalization of coagulation profile [23]. The addition of heparin in this study showed to have an increased risk of bleeding without any significant mortality benefit. The Kybersept RCT showed no mortality benefit of AT therapy over placebo [24]. However, a post-hoc analysis of this study revealed that the negative results for antithrombin were mainly due to co-administration of heparin, which caused an increased rate of bleeding [25].

Thrombomodulin

Thrombomodulin is a natural cofactor that primarily exerts its anticoagulant effect by activation of protein C. It also inhibits thrombus formation by suppressing thrombin activity [26, 27]. Soluble thrombomodulin (thromomodulin alfa, TM-α) is a recombinant version of thrombomodulin that was developed for the treatment of patients with DIC. A Phase 3 trial in Japan showed that TM-α has a better effect on coagulation profile and less bleeding manifestations than heparin [28]. The bleeding risk is less with TM-α as its activity depends on the amount of thrombin generated [29]. TM-α has been shown to have a beneficial effect on clinical outcomes and DIC parameters in few other trials [30]. A Phase 3 study is currently ongoing in US evaluating the efficacy of TM-α in patients suffering from sepsis induced DIC [31].

Activated Protein C

It is a natural anticoagulant with significant anti-inflammatory and anti-thrombotic roles in patients with sepsis. Based on the results of the Protein C Worldwide Evaluation in Severe Sepsis (PROWESS) trial conducted in 2001, recombinant human Activated Protein C (rhAPC), showed mortality reduction in patients with Sepsis related DIC [32]. An increase in use of rhAPC was seen following reports of proven benefits from several other studies [33, 34]. Later, the PROWESS-Shock trial failed to show any significant mortality benefit of rhAPC in patients with septic shock [35]. Hence, it is no longer recommended to use rhAPC in the treatment of DIC.

The Surviving Sepsis Campaign Guidelines (SSCG) also withdrew its recommendations to use rhAPC in 2012 after no proven efficacy of its use could be shown [36]. A recent meta-analysis concluded that rhAPC did provide a significant reduction in hospital mortality in patients with severe sepsis but at the same time showed a significant risk of bleeding in such patients [37]. The meta-analysis, however, also included retrospective studies along with the randomized controlled trials and therefore might have lead to the results being biased. A meta-analysis including only RCTs was published in 2007 and was recently updated after addition of another RCT [38]. The update, in line with the original results, failed to show any benefit of rhAPC in patients with severe sepsis and it concluded that rhAPC was associated with a higher risk of bleeding. Most recently, the report on a French multicenter double-blinded trial (The APROCCHSS trial) was published which concluded that rhAPC showed no benefit or harm in patients with severe septic shock [39].

Anti-Fibrinolytic Agents

Anti-fibrinolytic agents such as ε-aminocaproic acid or tranexamic acid are lysine-like drugs, which interfere with the formation of the plasmin from its precursor plasminogen by plasminogen activators. These drugs block the binding sites of the enzymes or plasminogen respectively and thus stop plasmin formation. The use of these agents is not usually preferred in DIC as it may lead to increase in thrombotic complications due to blockage of the fibrinolytic system [40]. An exception may be made in those rare cases where hyperfibrinolysis is predominant in the clinical picture such as in coagulopathy associated with acute promyelocytic leukemia (AML-M3) [41], massive postpartum hemorrhage [42] and acute coagulopathy of trauma [43].

The recommended dosage for use of tranexamic acid is 1g every 8 hours.

Synthetic Protease Inhibitors

Synthetic Protease Inhibitors such as Gabexate mesilate and Nafamstat act by blocking serine proteases, such as thrombin and plasmin, in the coagulation cascade and hence prevent activation of the coagulation factors. These agents have been used & evaluated for treatment of DIC accompanied by bleeding diathesis in Japan [44, 45]. However, there have been no RCTs that have evaluated their role in reduction of mortality or an improvement in the resolution rate in DIC. Further studies are warranted before it can be used.

Tissue Factor Pathway Inhibitor

Tissue factor pathway inhibitor (TFPI) is the principal endogenous inhibitor of the TF pathway. It acts by blocking both the initiation and the propagation of coagulation cascade [46]. It was thought of as a potential therapy in sepsis-induced DIC and initial results from animal studies looked very promising [47]. However, a large phase III trial of TFPI in humans did not show any benefit in mortality reduction [48].

Recombinant Human Factor VIIa

It acts by facilitating the activation of the extrinsic pathway of blood coagulation. There have been suggestions of its use in some patients with severe DIC-associated hemorrhage that is unresponsive to standard treatment [49]. However, there is a need for large RCTs to verify this fact before any conclusions can be drawn on its efficacy or safety in this setting.

Anti-Factor Xa Agents

Factor Xa is the most important factor in the coagulation cacase owing to its presence at the juncture of intrinsic and extrinsic pathways. Anti-Factor Xa agents act by direct or indirect inhibiton of this factor and therefore prevent the cleavage of prothrombin. One such agent, Fondaparinux has been recommended for DVT prophylaxis after orthopedic surgery [50], however there is very less evidence to support its use in critically ill patients.

DIC Treatment in Specific Conditions

Sepsis Induced DIC

The vicious cycle of inflammation and coagulation leads to the life threatening condition of DIC. Antibiotics and blood products is no doubt the most important part of the treatment but there iss more that can be done.

As discussed already, the PROWESS-SHOCK study removed rhAPC from the treatment pool of 'Septic DIC' completely and was withdrawn from the market despite of proven anti-inflammatory properties of rhAPC, as it did not show any 28 day mortality benefit but did increase bleeding risk (incidence being 5.6%)[35]. Earlier studies had shown some positive effect of APC on severe as well as mild form of the disease, and the decision of withdrawal of this treatment recommendation was solely based on a single study. Therefore, the possibility of re-introduction of APC in the market cannot be ruled out.

As mentioned above, the Kybersept failed to demonstrate any benefit of AT in septic DIC [24]. A recent non-randomized study in its Phase 4 has been able to demonstrate some benefit of AT when used at supplemental doses of 1500 IU/day or 3000 IU/day for three days. The important factors determining outcome in patients were pre-treatment AT levels, higher treatment dose (3000 IU/day), and young age. The study also demonstrated a lower overall risk of bleeding (6.5%) and serious bleeding (1.71%). If this study can show a statistically significant advantage in the future, it would be a good option to use AT at a dose of 3000 IU/day in septic DIC [51].

There is tissue factor upregulation in infection, but as already mentioned, many RCTs have failed to show any benefit of recombinant tissue factor inhibitor in patients of DIC [48]. Recombinant thrombomodulin has been recently considered for the treatment of septic DIC after a Phase 3 study in Japan showed some benefit on 28- day mortality, and reduced risk of bleeding [28]. As already mentioned, a Phase 3 study is underway in US to study efficacy of thrombomodulin in sepsis induced DIC [31].

Heparin and Heparinoids act through maximizing activity of AT III, although there is no reliable RCT to show its benefit in Septic DIC, a retrospective analysis showed mortality benefit of low dose heparin [52]. LMWH heparin is preferred over UH in patients with a tendency to bleed [13].

Obstetric DIC

Just like other forms of DIC, removal of offending factor is the most important intervention to put a halt on the ongoing disease process. The evacuation of uterus in case of retained placental or fetal parts and adequate volume resuscitation with support of vital organs is a wise step to get started [53]. The next step is to take care of the deranged coagulation. In cases of amniotic fluid embolism continuous leak in the system stimulates intravascular thrombosis. Low dose subcutaneous heparin can show an improvement in clinical and laboratory picture in 3-4 hours without significant increased risk of bleeding [54]. A switch to high dose intravenous heparin can be made if no improvement is seen with low subcutaneous doses. The risk of bleeding has to be considered always while treating with heparin. Other anti-coagulants like AT and rhAPC have shown some benefit but are not very well studied options.

Conclusion

In conclusion, the treatment options for DIC are quite a few owing to its varied etiology. The therapeutic approach to each patient depends on the etiology & clinical manifestations of DIC. Hence, it is safe to say that there is no single best answer when it comes to the question of treatment for DIC. Treatment of DIC needs to be individualized pertaining to signs and symptoms of the patient.

References

[1]   Levi M, Ten Cate H. Disseminated intravascular coagulation. *N. Engl. J. Med.* 1999;341(8):586-92. Epub 1999/08/19.

[2]   Levi M, Toh CH, Thachil J, Watson HG. Guidelines for the diagnosis and management of disseminated intravascular coagulation. British Committee for Standards in Haematology. *Br. J. Haematol.* 2009;145(1):24-33. Epub 2009/02/19.

[3]   Singh B, Hanson AC, Alhurani R, Wang S, Herasevich V, Cartin-Ceba R, et al. Trends in the incidence and outcomes of disseminated intravascular coagulation in critically ill patients (2004-2010): a population-based study. *Chest.* 2013;143(5):1235-42. Epub 2012/11/10.

[4]   Wada H, Asakura H, Okamoto K, Iba T, Uchiyama T, Kawasugi K, et al. Expert consensus for the treatment of disseminated intravascular coagulation in Japan. *Thromb Res.* 2010;125(1):6-11. Epub 2009/09/29.

[5]   Di Nisio M, Baudo F, Cosmi B, D'Angelo A, De Gasperi A, Malato A, et al. Diagnosis and treatment of disseminated intravascular coagulation: guidelines of the Italian Society for Haemostasis and Thrombosis (SISET). *Thromb Res.* 2012;129(5):e177-84. Epub 2011/09/21.

[6]   Kawasugi K, Wada H, Hatada T, Okamoto K, Uchiyama T, Kushimoto S, et al. Prospective evaluation of hemostatic abnormalities in overt DIC due to various underlying diseases. *Thromb Res.* 2011;128(2):186-90. Epub 2011/03/25.

[7]   Wada H, Thachil J, Di Nisio M, Mathew P, Kurosawa S, Gando S, et al. Guidance for diagnosis and treatment of DIC from harmonization of the recommendations from three guidelines. *J. Thromb Haemost.* 2013. Epub 2013/02/06.

[8]   Levi M, Opal SM. Coagulation abnormalities in critically ill patients. *Crit. Care.* 2006;10(4):222. Epub 2006/08/02.

[9]   Levi M. Disseminated intravascular coagulation: What's new? *Crit. Care Clin.* 2005;21(3):449-67. Epub 2005/07/05.

[10]   Franchini M, Lippi G, Manzato F. Recent acquisitions in the pathophysiology, diagnosis and treatment of disseminated intravascular coagulation. *Thromb J.* 2006;4:4. Epub 2006/03/01.

[11]   Hjort PF, Rapaport SI, Jorgensen L. Purpura Fulminans. Report of a Case Successfully Treated with Heparin and Hydrocortisone. Review of 50 Cases from the Literature. *Scand. J. Haematol.* 1964;1:169-92. Epub 1964/01/01.

[12]   Feinstein DI. Treatment of disseminated intravascular coagulation. *Semin. Thromb Hemost.* 1988;14(4):351-62. Epub 1988/10/01.

[13]   Sakuragawa N, Hasegawa H, Maki M, Nakagawa M, Nakashima M. Clinical evaluation of low-molecular-weight heparin (FR-860) on disseminated intravascular coagulation (DIC)--a multicenter co-

operative double-blind trial in comparison with heparin. *Thromb Res.* 1993;72(6):475-500. Epub 1993/12/15.

[14] Samama MM, Cohen AT, Darmon JY, Desjardins L, Eldor A, Janbon C, et al. A comparison of enoxaparin with placebo for the prevention of venous thromboembolism in acutely ill medical patients. Prophylaxis in Medical Patients with Enoxaparin Study Group. *N. Engl. J. Med.* 1999;341(11):793-800. Epub 1999/09/09.

[15] Patel R, Cook DJ, Meade MO, Griffith LE, Mehta G, Rocker GM, et al. Burden of illness in venous thromboembolism in critical care: a multicenter observational study. *J. Crit. Care.* 2005;20(4):341-7. Epub 2005/11/29.

[16] Cook DJ, Crowther MA, Meade MO, Douketis J. Prevalence, incidence, and risk factors for venous thromboembolism in medical-surgical intensive care unit patients. *J. Crit. Care.* 2005;20(4):309-13. Epub 2005/11/29.

[17] Feinstein DI. Diagnosis and management of disseminated intravascular coagulation: the role of heparin therapy. *Blood.* 1982;60(2):284-7. Epub 1982/08/01.

[18] [cited 2013 10th July]; Available from: http://www.uptodate.com/contents/clinical-features-diagnosis-and-treatment-of-disseminated-intravascular-coagulation-in-adults.

[19] Roemisch J, Gray E, Hoffmann JN, Wiedermann CJ. Antithrombin: a new look at the actions of a serine protease inhibitor. *Blood Coagul Fibrinolysis.* 2002;13(8):657-70. Epub 2002/11/21.

[20] Fourrier F, Chopin C, Huart JJ, Runge I, Caron C, Goudemand J. Double-blind, placebo-controlled trial of antithrombin III concentrates in septic shock with disseminated intravascular coagulation. *Chest.* 1993;104(3):882-8. Epub 1993/09/01.

[21] Mesters RM, Mannucci PM, Coppola R, Keller T, Ostermann H, Kienast J. Factor VIIa and antithrombin III activity during severe sepsis and septic shock in neutropenic patients. *Blood.* 1996;88(3):881-6. Epub 1996/08/01.

[22] Sivula M, Tallgren M, Pettila V. Modified score for disseminated intravascular coagulation in the critically ill. *Intensive Care Med.* 2005;31(9):1209-14. Epub 2005/06/17.

[23] Blauhut B, Kramar H, Vinazzer H, Bergmann H. Substitution of antithrombin III in shock and DIC: a randomized study. *Thromb Res.* 1985;39(1):81-9. Epub 1985/07/01.

[24] Warren BL, Eid A, Singer P, Pillay SS, Carl P, Novak I, et al. Caring for the critically ill patient. High-dose antithrombin III in severe sepsis: a randomized controlled trial. *JAMA.* 2001;286(15):1869-78. Epub 2001/10/26.

[25] Kienast J, Juers M, Wiedermann CJ, Hoffmann JN, Ostermann H, Strauss R, et al. Treatment effects of high-dose antithrombin without concomitant heparin in patients with severe sepsis with or without disseminated intravascular coagulation. *J. Thromb Haemost.* 2006;4(1):90-7. Epub 2006/01/18.

[26] Mohri M, Sugimoto E, Sata M, Asano T. The inhibitory effect of recombinant human soluble thrombomodulin on initiation and extension of coagulation--a comparison with other anticoagulants. *Thromb Haemost.* 1999;82(6):1687-93. Epub 1999/12/29.

[27] Maruyama I. Recombinant thrombomodulin and activated protein C in the treatment of disseminated intravascular coagulation. *Thromb Haemost.* 1999;82(2):718-21. Epub 1999/12/22.

[28] Saito H, Maruyama I, Shimazaki S, Yamamoto Y, Aikawa N, Ohno R, et al. Efficacy and safety of recombinant human soluble thrombomodulin (ART-123) in disseminated intravascular coagulation: results of a phase III, randomized, double-blind clinical trial. *J. Thromb Haemost.* 2007;5(1):31-41. Epub 2006/10/25.

[29] Ito T, Maruyama I. Thrombomodulin: protectorate God of the vasculature in thrombosis and inflammation. *J. Thromb Haemost.* 2011;9 Suppl 1:168-73. Epub 2011/08/04.

[30] Yamakawa K, Fujimi S, Mohri T, Matsuda H, Nakamori Y, Hirose T, et al. Treatment effects of recombinant human soluble thrombomodulin in patients with severe sepsis: a historical control study. *Crit. Care.* 2011;15(3):R123. Epub 2011/05/17.

[31] Available from: http://clinicaltrials.gov/ct2/show/nct01598831? term=ART-123&rank=2.

[32] Bernard GR, Vincent JL, Laterre PF, LaRosa SP, Dhainaut JF, Lopez-Rodriguez A, et al. Efficacy and safety of recombinant human activated protein C for severe sepsis. *N. Engl. J. Med.* 2001;344(10):699-709. Epub 2001/03/10.

[33] Dhainaut JF, Yan SB, Joyce DE, Pettila V, Basson B, Brandt JT, et al. Treatment effects of drotrecogin alfa (activated) in patients with severe sepsis with or without overt disseminated intravascular coagulation. *J. Thromb Haemost.* 2004;2(11):1924-33. Epub 2004/11/20.

[34] de Pont AC, Bakhtiari K, Hutten BA, de Jonge E, Vroom MB, Meijers JC, et al. Recombinant human activated protein C resets thrombin generation in patients with severe sepsis - a case control study. *Crit. Care.* 2005;9(5):R490-7. Epub 2005/11/10.

[35] Ranieri VM, Thompson BT, Barie PS, Dhainaut JF, Douglas IS, Finfer S, et al. Drotrecogin alfa (activated) in adults with septic shock. *N. Engl. J. Med.* 2012;366(22):2055-64. Epub 2012/05/24.

[36] Green J, Adams J, Panacek E, Albertson T. The 2012 Surviving Sepsis Campaign: Management of Severe Sepsis and Septic Shock—An Update on the Guidelines for Initial Therapy. Current Emergency and Hospital Medicine Reports. 2013:1-18.

[37] Kalil AC, LaRosa SP. Effectiveness and safety of drotrecogin alfa (activated) for severe sepsis: a meta-analysis and metaregression. *Lancet Infect Dis.* 2012;12(9):678-86. Epub 2012/07/20.

[38] Marti-Carvajal AJ, Sola I, Gluud C, Lathyris D, Cardona AF. Human recombinant protein C for severe sepsis and septic shock in adult and paediatric patients. *Cochrane Database Syst. Rev.* 2012;12:CD004388. Epub 2012/12/14.

[39] Annane D, Timsit JF, Megarbane B, Martin C, Misset B, Mourvillier B, et al. Recombinant human activated protein C for adults with septic shock: a randomized controlled trial. *Am. J. Respir. Crit. Care Med.* 2013;187(10):1091-7. Epub 2013/03/26.

[40] Ratnoff OD. Epsilon aminocaproic acid--a dangerous weapon. *N. Engl. J. Med.* 1969;280(20):1124-5. Epub 1969/05/15.

[41] de la Serna J, Montesinos P, Vellenga E, Rayon C, Parody R, Leon A, et al. Causes and prognostic factors of remission induction failure in patients with acute promyelocytic leukemia treated with all-trans retinoic acid and idarubicin. *Blood.* 2008;111(7):3395-402. Epub 2008/01/16.

[42] Ducloy-Bouthors AS, Jude B, Duhamel A, Broisin F, Huissoud C, Keita-Meyer H, et al. High-dose tranexamic acid reduces blood loss in postpartum haemorrhage. *Crit. Care.* 2011;15(2):R117. Epub 2011/04/19.

[43] Shakur H, Roberts I, Bautista R, Caballero J, Coats T, Dewan Y, et al. Effects of tranexamic acid on death, vascular occlusive events, and blood transfusion in trauma patients with significant haemorrhage (CRASH-2): a randomised, placebo-controlled trial. *Lancet.* 2010;376(9734):23-32. Epub 2010/06/18.

[44] Umeki S, Adachi M, Watanabe M, Yaji S, Soejima R. Gabexate as a therapy for disseminated intravascular coagulation. *Arch. Intern Med.* 1988;148(6):1409-12. Epub 1988/06/01.

[45] Okamura T, Niho Y, Itoga T, Chiba S, Miyake M, Kotsuru M, et al. Treatment of disseminated intravascular coagulation and its prodromal stage with gabaxate mesilate (FOY): a multi-center trial. *Acta Haematol.* 1993;90(3):120-4. Epub 1993/01/01.

[46] Kato H. Regulation of functions of vascular wall cells by tissue factor pathway inhibitor: basic and clinical aspects. *Arterioscler Thromb Vasc. Biol.* 2002;22(4):539-48. Epub 2002/04/16.

[47] Abraham E. Tissue factor inhibition and clinical trial results of tissue factor pathway inhibitor in sepsis. *Crit. Care Med.* 2000;28(9 Suppl):S31-3. Epub 2000/09/28.

[48] Abraham E, Reinhart K, Opal S, Demeyer I, Doig C, Rodriguez AL, et al. Efficacy and safety of tifacogin (recombinant tissue factor pathway inhibitor) in severe sepsis: a randomized controlled trial. *JAMA.* 2003;290(2):238-47. Epub 2003/07/10.

[49] Franchini M, Manzato F, Salvagno GL, Lippi G. Potential role of recombinant activated factor VII for the treatment of severe bleeding associated with disseminated intravascular coagulation: a systematic review. *Blood Coagul Fibrinolysis.* 2007;18(7):589-93. Epub 2007/09/25.

[50] Turpie AG, Bauer KA, Eriksson BI, Lassen MR. Fondaparinux vs enoxaparin for the prevention of venous thromboembolism in major orthopedic surgery: a meta-analysis of 4 randomized double-blind studies. *Arch. Intern Med.* 2002;162(16):1833-40. Epub 2002/08/28.

[51] Iba T, Saito D, Wada H, Asakura H. Efficacy and bleeding risk of antithrombin supplementation in septic disseminated intravascular coagulation: a prospective multicenter survey. *Thromb Res.* 2012;130(3):e129-33. Epub 2012/05/01.

[52] Polderman KH, Girbes AR. Drug intervention trials in sepsis: divergent results. *Lancet.* 2004;363(9422):1721-3. Epub 2004/05/26.

[53] Eskes TK. Abruptio placentae. A "classic" dedicated to Elizabeth Ramsey. *Eur. J. Obstet. Gynecol. Reprod. Biol.* 1997;75(1):63-70. Epub 1998/02/03.

[54] Bonnar J. Massive obstetric haemorrhage. *Baillieres Best Pract. Res. Clin. Obstet. Gynaecol.* 2000;14(1):1-18. Epub 2000/05/02.

Index

B

C

D

E

F

G

H

R

S